Tell Me What to Eat If I Suffer From Heart Disease

Nutrition You Can Live With

By Elaine Magee, MPH RD

A division of The Career Press, Inc.

Franklin Lakes, NJ

TELL ME WHAT TO EAT IF I SUFFER FROM HEART DISEASE
EDITED BY NICOLE DEFELICE

WITHDRAWN FROM
DÚN LAOGHAIRE-RATHDOWN COUNTY
LIBRARY STOCK

TYPESET BY DIANA GHAZZAWI

Cover design by Lucia Rossman / DigiDog Design
Printed in the U.S.A. by Courier

To order this title, please call toll-free 1-800-CAREER-1 (NJ and Canada: 201-848-0310) to order using VISA or MasterCard, or for further information on books from Career Press.

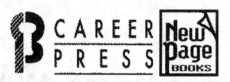

The Career Press, Inc., 3 Tice Road, PO Box 687,
Franklin Lakes, NJ 07417
www.careerpress.com
www.newpagebooks.com

Library of Congress Cataloging-in-Publication Data
Magee, Elaine.
    Tell me what to eat if I suffer from heart disease : nutrition you can live with / by Elaine Magee.
        p. cm.
    ISBN 978-1-60163-097-1
    1. Heart--Diseases--Diet therapy. I. Title.

RC684.D5M34 2010
616.1'20654--dc22

                                                                2009045349

Contents

Introduction

If you bought this book, maybe it's because you've suffered a heart attack or have been told you have heart disease. Perhaps you have high blood cholesterol or high blood pressure, or are at high risk for heart disease. This book is for all of you.

It may not seem like it, but there has never been a better time to be in your position. Treatments for heart disease, discoveries related to reversing heart disease, advances in medication, and the surgical options are all much better than even 10 years ago.

The typical American diet works against our genetics, leading most of us down a path toward assorted dangerous health issues such as heart disease and stroke. For example, the average diet embraces the tempting trifecta of fat, sugar, and salt—a combination that some experts say encourages overeating and a dulling of our natural ability to compensate for extra calories. Think of some favorite American foods—they all have a combination of fat, sugar, and/or salt (sodium):

- French fries (fat and salt)
- Potato chips (fat and salt)

- Chocolate (fat, sugar, and a hint of salt)
- Cheeseburgers (fat and salt)
- Ice cream and milk shakes (fat and sugar)
- Pizza (fat and salt)
- Snack cakes and cookies (fat and sugar)
- Bacon (fat and salt)

The same powerful changes you'll need to make to turn around the risk for heart disease will also reduce the risk of other chronic illnesses. The underlying cause of both heart disease and stroke is atherosclerosis (plaque deposits in our arteries), and one of the triggers of atherosclerosis is inflammation in the body. So the lifestyle changes we suggest throughout this book will have anti-inflammation and anti-plaquing actions in the body.

You've probably heard this before: Heart disease is the number-one killer of both men and women. You would think this affects only older adults, but more than 151,000 Americans who died of cardiovascular diseases in 2005 were younger than age 65.

This book will help:

- If you are at low risk for having a heart attack. A healthy lifestyle (balanced diet, daily exercise, and not smoking) will help protect you for the future.
- If you have some of the risk factors for heart disease, but are in the early stages. You should be motivated to make specific lifestyle and diet changes that will help reduce your personal risk factors.
- If you have heart disease or are at high risk for having a heart attack. Exercise and healthful eating are vital, along with controlling blood pressure, blood lipids, blood sugar, and using appropriate medications to keep the risk for future heart and stroke events as low as possible.

In the past few years, there have been hundreds of new discoveries related to the treatment and prevention of heart disease. This book incorporates much of this new information and gives you practical tips for cooking, shopping, and eating out that will slow, stop, and even reverse heart disease.

You will learn about the 10 food steps toward a diet that will curb inflammation and atherosclerosis in the body. You will also discover:

- Heart disease superfoods—specific foods that help protect your heart and arteries and should be eaten almost every day.

- The 10 things cardiologists really want you to know after you've been diagnosed with heart disease.

- Five things you can do today to improve your blood pressure and stroke risk tomorrow.

- How to lose weight without dieting, and why your hip and waist measurements are more important than what you weigh.

- Six steps that could prevent more than 27 million heart attacks nationwide.

- How the "Smart Heart Food Journal"—a blank form that you use each day—could turn your lifestyle around.

Choose to feel better. Choose to make the types of changes that will not only help your heart, but will help you lose weight, and will help prevent diseases such as stroke, diabetes, and cancer.

Chapter 1

The Who, What, Where, Why, and How of Heart Disease

They're costly and they're common. Here's the irony—heart disease and stroke are among the most widespread and costly health problems in America, and yet they are also among the most preventable diseases. The projected cost for heart disease and stroke in the United States for 2009 was more than $475 billion, according to the Centers for Disease Control and Prevention. And this bottom-line cost (including healthcare expenditures and lost productivity) will only go higher, given that baby boomers are mostly 50 and over.

Here are some fast statistics on heart disease and stroke—the number-one and number-three killers—in the United States:

- More than one in three adults (80 million) live with one or more types of cardiovascular disease.
- Each year, there are an estimated 935,000 heart attacks and 795,000 strokes.
- Americans make more than 72 million doctor visits every year for treatment and management of cardiovascular diseases.

- More than 7 million hospitalizations occur each year because of cardiovascular diseases. ("Heart Disease and Stroke Pevention: Addressing the Nation's Leading Killers." *Centers for Disease Control and Prevention*)

Here's a sobering fact: By the time we reach 20, just about all of us have some amount of atherosclerosis in our arteries. Why is that important? The underlying issue in heart disease and stroke is the accumulation of atherosclerotic plaque (fatty deposits in the inner lining of arteries) triggered in part by inflammation in the body.

Atherosclerosis starts with an insult or injury to the delicate endothelium (the inner lining of arteries). Common insults include high blood pressure, high blood sugar, a barrage of inflammatory signals from excess body fat, damage from turbulent blood flow, noxious chemicals from cigarette smoke, and too much fat or cholesterol in the bloodstream.

The January 2009 issue of the *Harvard Heart Letter* described the process of atherosclerosis plaque and arterial injury: "The damage causes some cells in the endothelium to become sticky. Like flypaper, they snare passing white blood cells and entice them to burrow into the lining. These white blood cells stir up a ferment of inflammatory cells and signals. Over time, a new matrix of tissue begins to form. It attracts cholesterol-carrying LDL particles innocently circulating through the blood. As LDL cholesterol slips inside cells, the cells' highly reactive contents oxidize it. Circulating white blood cells sense this change as a threat to the body. They seek out the oxidized LDL and gorge on it. As they fill up and begin to die, they give off more inflammatory signals, perpetuating and accelerating the cycle. The activity leads to gooey pools of plaque embedded here and there in the endothelium. Each one is separated from the bloodstream by a thin cap."

What cardiologists now realize is that the danger of plaque breaking open often comes from soft plaque with a thin cap that barely pokes into the artery and isn't easily detected by an angiogram or stress test. A heart attack can occur when plaque breaks open and causes the body to produce a clot that fills the artery and completely blocks blood flow to part of the heart muscle.

Other names for a heart attack include:

- Myocardial infarction
- Coronary thrombosis (thrombosis is the formation of one or more clots that may partially or completely block the coronary artery)
- Coronary occlusion (occlusion is when something is obstructing or blocking the coronary artery)

A stroke can occur when the plaque ruptures in an artery going to the brain. An ischemic stroke (the most common kind of stroke) can occur when the rupturing plaque happens somewhere else in the body and the clot breaks loose and travels to the brain.

What's an Aneurysm?

An aneurysm is a ballooning of a weakened region of a blood vessel. If left untreated, it will continue to weaken until it ruptures. Aneurysms are often caused, or made worse, by high blood pressure. If they burst in the brain, they cause a hemorrhagic stroke. A cerebral hemorrhage occurs when a diseased artery in the brain bursts, flooding the surrounding tissue with blood.

What's a TIA?

TIA stands for transient ischemic attacks. They are minor strokes that come with the warning signs of a stroke, but the blood clot occurs for a short time and tends to resolve itself. Obviously having a TIA is an indicator that a major stroke is very likely in the near future.

Know the Signs— It Could Save Your Life

Do you know the warning signs for a heart attack or stroke? Chest pain or pressure is the most common symptom of a heart attack. But keep in mind that women are more likely than men to experience symptoms other than chest pain.

Signs and Symptoms of a Heart Attack

(W = symptoms that are more likely to occur in women)

- Chest discomfort that may feel like pressure, squeezing, fullness, or pain and may last for more than a few minutes, or may come and go.
- Shortness of breath, which may or may not go along with chest pain.
- Discomfort in other parts of the upper body, including one or both arms, the back, neck, jaw, or stomach.
- Breaking out in a cold sweat.
- Indigestion or gas-like pain or nausea. (W)
- Unexplained dizziness, weakness, or fatigue. (W)
- Discomfort or pain between the shoulder blades. (W)
- Racing or fluttering heart.
- A hot or flushed feeling.
- Recurring chest discomfort. (W)
- Sense of impending doom. (W)

Signs and Symptoms of a Stroke

(The following symptoms may become more noticeable over time.)

- Sudden numbness or weakness in the face, arm, or leg, especially on one side of the body.
- Sudden confusion or trouble speaking or understanding.
- Sudden vision problem in one or both eyes.
- Sudden dimming of vision, especially in one eye.
- Sudden dizziness, difficulty walking, loss of balance or coordination (possibly accompanied by vomiting, nausea, fever, hiccups, or trouble swallowing).
- Sudden, severe headache with no known cause.
- Brief loss of consciousness.

What Is Cardiac Arrest?

Cardiac arrest is the sudden, complete loss of heart function. Brain death and permanent death start to occur in just four to six minutes after someone goes into cardiac arrest. It happens in people who may or may not have been diagnosed with heart disease. Irregular heart rhythm (arrhythmia) causes the heart to suddenly stop beating. Sometimes electrical impulses in the diseased heart become rapid (ventricular tachycardia), chaotic (ventricular fibrillation), or both. Someone can be brought out of cardiac arrest if treated within a few minutes with an electric shock (defibrillation) to the heart, which helps restore the normal heartbeat. You've undoubtedly seen this happen on hospital television shows. With every minute that goes by, the person's chance of surviving reduces by 10 percent.

Signs of Cardiac Arrest

- Sudden collapse with no responsiveness.
- Absence of normal breathing.

What Is Heart Failure?

Heart failure can result when your heart isn't pumping blood as well as it should, which prevents the other organs from getting enough blood. Blood flowing out of the heart slows down, and blood returning to the heart through the veins backs up, causing congestion (with too much fluid accumulating) in the body tissues. See a doctor immediately if you notice any of the warning signs.

Heart failure in people 50 years of age or younger is much more common among African Americans than any other ethnicity. In general, if certain risk factors of heart failure appeared before you were 35 years of age, such as high blood pressure, obesity, and systolic dysfunction (which would have been discovered during an echocardiogram), you could be at a higher risk for heart failure within the next 10 years. For example, 75 percent of people who went on to have heart failure developed hypertension by the time they were 40 years old, according to a new study.

Signs of Heart Failure
(or Congestive Heart Failure)

- Swelling in the feet, ankles, and legs (edema), which is most common, but it can happen in other parts of the body, also.
- Fluid buildup in the lungs (pulmonary congestion), causing shortness of breath, especially when you are lying down. (*New England Journal of Medicine* 360 (2009): 1179–1190)

If you think you are having a heart attack or stroke, act quickly by calling 911 or your local emergency number. Transportation by ambulance is recommended because medical care can begin right away. Don't delay, because every minute counts. If you are having a heart attack, survival rates improve by 50 percent if you get medical care within an hour.

Six Steps to Prevent 27 Million Heart Attacks

Current scientific evidence shows that taking these six steps today will prevent more than 27 million heart attacks and about 10 million strokes throughout the next 30 years. And that's just in the United States. According to the American Heart Association, the six steps that could very well save and prolong your life are:

1. Quit smoking.
2. Get your body mass index (BMI) out of the "obese" range (BMI of 30 or greater).
3. Get your LDL ("bad" cholesterol) under control (at or below 70mg/dL is the target range).
4. Get your blood pressure into the normal range (120/80 is healthy).
5. Get your blood sugar under control, especially if you have diabetes (fasting blood glucose is 70-99 mg/dL; two hours after eating is 70-145 mg/dL).
6. Take aspirin if your doctor tells you to because of heart disease risk.

There are a few more steps I would add to this list to help you accomplish steps 2 through 5 and help cut your risk by 92 percent. They are: Eat a heart-smart diet emphasizing high-nutrient, low-calorie foods with smart carbs, smart fats, and lean protein; get active with regular exercise almost every day (about 40 minutes);

drink only a moderate amount of alcohol; keep your waist trimmer than your hips; and decrease the stress and anxiety in your life.

Heart disease kills close to half a million women each year, more than all cancers combined. Some new data suggests that women may be more likely than men to need a heart-healthy lifestyle makeover if premature heart attacks run in their families (meaning a parent or sibling who has had a heart attack before age 50 for men or 55 for women).

In a Swedish study of postmenopausal women, heart attacks were 92 percent less likely in the women who practiced all of these heart-healthy habits compared with the women who did none of them. Each habit contributes individually to the reduction in risk. For example, women who practiced the first two habits were 57 percent less likely to have a heart attack than other women. (Akesson A. *Archives of Internal Medicine* 167 (2007): 2122–2127.)

Another study tracked more than 114,000 men and women with the average age of 50 between 1986 and 2002. Researchers found that having a healthy lifestyle helped cut the risk of ischemic stroke by 80 percent. In addition to not smoking and watching alcohol intake, these other habits contributed to the lowest risk: a body mass index of less than 25, moderate to vigorous activity for 30 minutes or more daily, and a diet low in "bad" fats and rich in vegetables, fruits, and lean protein such as chicken and fish, fiber, nuts, and beans. (*American Stroke Association*)

The 10 Things Cardiologists Really Want You to Know

Cardiologists are specialists in heart conditions, which include abnormal heart rhythms, heart attacks, coronary artery disease, congenital heart defects, and disease of the heart valves. These are the doctors you usually develop a close relationship with once you have signs of heart disease.

Cardiologists use an assortment of tests and tools to study heart conditions, including:

- Cardiac stress test: A test of heart function after a standardized amount of exertion.

- Exercise stress echo: This involves exercising on a treadmill or stationary bicycle while you and your heart are closely monitored.

- Biopsy: A tiny piece of heart tissue is removed and studied.

- Echocardiogram (often called "echo"): This is a graphic outline of the heart's movement, valves, and chambers using high-frequency sound waves that come from a handheld wand placed on your chest. An echo is often combined with Doppler ultrasound and color Doppler to evaluate blood flow across the heart's valves.

- Electrocardiogram (EKG or ECG): A test that records on graph paper the electrical activity of the heart via small electrode patches attached to the skin. An EKG helps a physician determine the causes of abnormal heartbeat or detect heart damage.

- Angiography: An invasive imaging procedure that usually involves inserting a catheter into an artery leading to the heart muscle or brain and injecting a radioactive tracer into the bloodstream. This test is used to determine if there is fatty buildup or plaque in the arteries that is causing narrowing. Coronary angiography is also called cardiac catheterization.

Because cardiologists are on the front lines of heart disease treatment, I wanted to know what they want you to know if you've been diagnosed with heart disease. The following is based on interviews with a few wonderful, passionate cardiologists.

1. There's no room for smoking (or secondhand smoke).

If you are a smoker, you have to quit. Not smoking is the number-one priority for many cardiologists—there is no room for it when you have heart disease. "Smoking makes any plaque in your arteries that are unstable more unstable," says Dr. Matthew DeVane, author of *Heart Smart* and a cardiologist with Cardiovascular Consulting Group in Walnut Creek, California. Here's what else tobacco does:

- The chemicals in tobacco smoke increase the buildup of plaque in artery walls and promote the development of blood clots that cause heart attacks.

- Smoking increases the risk of coronary heart disease.

- Smoking enhances the detrimental effect of other risk factors such as diabetes, high blood pressure, and high cholesterol.

- Smokers have more than twice the risk of having a heart attack compared to nonsmokers.

- Exposure to tobacco smoke (including cigar, pipe, or any kind of secondhand smoke) increases your chance of coronary heart disease.

And yet nearly one out of every five Americans is still smoking cigarettes—that's 43.4 million Americans. (The percentage of smokers has been going down steadily since the mid-1960s, when about 42 percent of American adults smoked.)

When people try to quit smoking alone, without help, the success rate of staying smoke-free is only about 5 percent. So work with your doctor to get all the help you can to stop smoking for good. Cardiologists say it may take several attempts to permanently kick the habit, but it's worth it. The benefits for those who quit are huge, including dramatically reducing the risk of cardiovascular disease and lung cancer.

2. You are probably not exercising enough.

The second most important step is to get exercise almost every day. Most people who think they are exercising enough really aren't. They might walk 30 minutes twice a week, but if they want to see big changes, they are going to have to do more, such as aerobic exercise for 45 to 60 minutes most days. DeVane often tells his patients to walk faster, walk longer, and/or add hand weights. For those who need to lose weight, DeVane says it takes exercising 60 to 90 minutes to burn enough calories to lose weight when you are eating around 2,000 calories a day.

3. The first month is critical.

The first month after having a first heart event or being diagnosed with heart disease is a precious small window of opportunity. This is when newly diagnosed patients are open and willing (or scared enough) to make significant lifestyle changes.

4. Set specific goals for yourself.

Don't just set the goal to exercise more. Be more specific. Set the goal to exercise a certain number of days each week or to reach 10,000 steps a day on your pedometer. If you want to set a goal for losing weight, you might be better off setting the goal to lose a certain amount of inches around your waist and to accomplish this with lifestyle changes that you can live with instead of dieting.

5. Big portions are a big barrier to weight-loss success.

Several of the cardiologists I interviewed say eating smaller portions can help people trim extra calories from their daily totals. Most agree that Americans have grown so accustomed to buying and consuming huge portions of food and beverages that we now think it's normal. Dr. Neal White, MD, director of the Cardiac Catheterization Lab for the San Ramon Regional Medical Center in Northern California, recommends that his patients keep a food diary. "One of the biggest benefits," he says, "is that people often realize they were eating or drinking more than they thought they were." For more on how to lose weight without dieting and a sample food journal, see Chapter 3.

6. If you drink alcohol, you are most likely drinking too much.

DeVane never recommends alcohol to patients who don't already drink. He believes the benefits aren't so great that you need to start drinking. What about the patients who do drink alcohol? "Most of them are drinking too much," he says. He strongly recommends that his patients who do drink keep it moderate: no more than one drink a day for women, and no more than two drinks a day for men. If you are overweight, you should move away from alcohol because it adds extra calories. And even though health benefits are associated with a moderate intake of alcohol, it's really difficult for some people to stop at one glass of wine per day. Alcohol can drive up serum triglycerides too, particularly for those who already have higher levels of serum triglycerides.

7. Today's medications offer great options.

"The medications that we have now are so safe and so strong," says DeVane, who believes in the powerful combination of taking appropriate medications to control heart disease and its risk factors, making healthful lifestyle changes, and exercising regularly. He stresses the importance of following up with your appointments and doing the laboratory work as requested by your doctor.

8. What you do next is vitally important.

If you have heart disease or high blood pressure, or have had a heart attack, what you do about the environmental factors in your life helps determine what happens next, according to White. "The people who tend to do the best after a cardiovascular event are the ones who lose weight," he says. "Most heart disease patients can stand to lose 5 to 10 pounds and up to 20 pounds," he adds.

9. Tell your cardiologist if you have any symptoms in your chest.

After you've had one cardiovascular event or been diagnosed with heart disease, you need to bring any symptoms happening in your chest to the attention of your cardiologist immediately. They could occur while you are exerting yourself during certain activities, such as mowing the lawn, running on the treadmill, or playing golf.

10. Women need to remember that heart disease is their number-one killer.

"Women overall tend to focus on cancer as the disease to prevent," explains White, "but it's sudden death from heart disease that actually kills more women year after year."

Beyond Diet

More than just lifestyle habits can hurt your heart. Let's look at some of those.

A bad marriage or negative relationships with close friends is on the list. If you are in a bad or negative relationship, you are 34 percent more likely to have a coronary event in the next decade or so, suggests a study that followed more than 9,000 British male and female civil servants for 12 years. The increase in risk dropped to 25 percent, however, after the researchers took into account other variables that could contribute to heart disease, such as depression. This applied not only to married men and women, but also to those who were unmarried but had negative relationships with close friends. Researchers suspect that negative relationships can activate emotional responses such as depression or hostility, which in turn might hurt the heart over time. (*Archives of Internal Medicine* 167(2007): 1951–1957.)

Depression, hostility, and anger are considered emotional risk factors to many heart experts. Recent studies have found that this link to heart disease holds solid, even when other heart disease risk factors are considered. When researchers pooled data from 44 studies worldwide, they found that chronically angry or hostile adults with no history of heart disease might be 19 percent more likely to develop heart disease. What happens once you have heart disease? Angry or hostile heart disease patients may be 24 percent more likely than other heart patients to have a poor prognosis.

A recent study raised questions about a possible link between antidepressant use and the risk of sudden cardiac death, and some antidepressants (tricyclic antidepressants) are thought to have possible effects on cardiac arrhythmias. More needs to be known about all of this, but if you are taking antidepressants or considering them, it's worth discussing these possible issues with your doctor, psychiatrist, or cardiologist.

(Whang, W., et al. "Depression and Risk of Sudden Cardiac Death and Coronary Heart Disease in Women" and Chida, Y., et al "The Association of Anger and Hostility with Future Coronary Heart Disease." *Journal of the American College of Cardiology.* 17 Mar 2009.)

A Look Inside Your Mouth

How clean is your mouth? Believe it or not, the answer to that question might help or hurt your heart. The higher the amount of two types of oral bacteria (Tannerella Forsynthesis and Preventella Intermedia)—and in particular, the higher the total number of bacteria in the mouth—the higher the risk of heart attack, a University of Buffalo study shows.

In the study, samples of dental plaque were collected from 12 sites in the gums of two groups: men and women who suffered a heart attack, and men and women who were free of heart trouble. Dental plaque samples were telling, because bacteria tend to adhere to it in the mouth. The researchers found that an increase in the number of periodontal bacteria increased the odds of having a heart attack. More research needs to be done to understand exactly what's at play here, but we should all want to keep the amount of oral bacteria low anyway, right?

What's the best way to improve oral health? Brush twice daily, floss daily, and use mouthwash "as an adjunct to the brushing and flossing," says Karen Falkner, PhD, associate director for Research Studies, Periodontal Disease Center, University of Buffalo. (International Association of Dental Research, Apr 2009.)

Air Pollution

There is growing evidence that an increase in air pollution—including smoke from cigarettes, cooking oil, and wood—is associated with an increase in heart attacks and deaths.

- A study of six U.S. cities found that people died earlier when they lived in cities with higher pollution levels; a majority of those deaths were due to heart disease.

- A study of 250 metropolitan areas around the world noted that a spike in air pollution is followed by a spike in heart attacks.

- The risk of heart attack increases as the time spent in traffic the previous day increases.

It makes sense that living in an area with significant air pollution is going to hurt your lungs and the first place the air goes is your lungs. But experts now know that air pollution has short-term and long-term toxic effects on the heart and blood vessels. A recent study by the University of Kentucky found that even small doses of secondhand smoke (from tobacco, cooking oil, or wood) affected cardiovascular function in men and women exposed for as little as 10 minutes. ("Smoke from cigarettes, cooking oil, wood, shift male cardiovascular system into overdrive." *American Physiological Society.* press release. 17 Apr 2009.)

There are several ways that smoke and pollution can hurt the heart. One toxic class of chemicals, called aldehydes, are found in most forms of smoke such as cigarettes and car exhaust, and increase blood cholesterol levels and activate enzymes that cause plaque in the blood vessels to rupture. When plaque ruptures, a blood clot can form, which may lead to an artery blockage, and heart attack.

Fine and ultrafine particles in smoke and pollution that get into the lungs and find their way into the blood vessels can cause a very rapid increase in blood pressure (within 15 minutes), according to Robert Brook, MD, Assistant Professor of Internal Medicine with the University of Michigan. The blood vessels then attack the foreign matter (the pollutants) by producing an inflammatory response, which can set off a cascade of physiological events that can be harmful to blood vessels and the cardiovascular system.

According to Robert Kloner, MD, PhD, director of Research at the Heart Institute of the Good Samaritan Hospital, research suggests that ultrafine air pollutants (like those coming from car exhaust) may get into the lungs and gain entrance to the bloodstream. Normally, the upper airway filters out the larger particles that are in smog and other air pollutants before they can cause a problem.

When the Heart Institute studied what happens when hearts are directly exposed to ultrafine air pollutants, researchers discovered an immediate decrease in coronary blood flow, a decrease in the heart's pumping function, and an increase in the development of arrhythmias—three things that you do not want happening. According to Z. Simkhovich, MD, PhD, a senior research associate at the Heart Institute, air pollution can be dangerous even at levels that are within the accepted air quality standards.

The elderly and patients who have already been diagnosed with heart disease or diabetes (which tends to increase damage to blood vessels) are particularly vulnerable to the cardiovascular effects of air pollution.

So what should you do if you are in one of these groups, or if you just want to reduce your exposure to air pollution? During times when air quality is bad or borderline bad, exercise indoors, because indoor air is filtered. If you exercise outdoors, do so when pollutants are at lower levels. Avoid being out in peak traffic times as much as possible. And during the winter, limit your exposure to fireplace smoke.

Get Some Sleep!

A small study of 12 young, healthy men found that getting only four hours of sleep two nights in a row led to an increase in the hunger hormone, ghrelin, and increased hunger and appetite, and a decrease in the anti-hunger hormone, leptin, compared to sleeping 10 hours a night for two nights.

Short-term sleep deprivation studies have suggested that markers of inflammation (measured in the blood) tend to be elevated in people who are sleep-deprived. People who sleep less than five hours a night tend to have an increased risk of death from cardiovascular disease, have lower mental and physical health scores, and are more likely to smoke and have higher systolic blood pressure. But when it comes to sleep, a whole lot more might not be better, either. Men and women sleeping nine hours or more tend to be more likely to have decreased physical health scores. Looks like seven to eight hours a night is just right.

Trials have shown that many people could get to sleep a little sooner if they used relaxation techniques that helped them "switch off" at bedtime. These are the habits that some sleep experts say might help people sleep better:

- Only go to bed when you are tired and ready to go to sleep.
- Reading and watching TV in bed actually makes it harder to fall asleep.
- If you cannot sleep, it is actually better for you to get out of bed and do something else rather than focus on trying to sleep.
- Getting up at the same time every morning.
- If you are having issues with insomnia, napping during the day could be making it harder for you to sleep at night.
- Drinking caffeinated beverages and alcohol in the evening isn't going to help your sleep situation. It's not just caffeine keeping people up; alcohol is one of the major causes of a bad night's sleep. (Spiegel, et al. "Brief Communication: Sleep Curtailment in Healthy Young Men Is Associated with Decreased Leptin Levels, Elevated Ghrelin Levels, and

Increased Hunger and Appetite." *Annals of Internal Medicine* 141.11 (2004): 846–850.)

People who have obstructive sleep apnea may have their sleep interrupted several times a night when the upper airway becomes completely or partially blocked. A study including 92 people who had recently had a heart attack found that the patients with obstructive sleep apnea were six times more likely to have had their heart attack between midnight and 6 a.m. than during the rest of the day. Some researchers suspect that obstructive sleep apnea may be a trigger for heart attacks, but more research needs to be done to see if sleep apnea treatment translates into a reduced risk for heart attacks, especially at night. (*Journal of the American College of Cardiology* 52 (2008): 343–346.)

Plastic Bottle Chemicals

BPA—bisphenol A—is used to make hard clear plastic and can be found in many food product containers as well. It is an environmental pollutant linked to neurological defects, diabetes, and breast and prostate cancer and thought to have estrogen activity in the body. To this list of potential harmful effects, we add the possible link to an increased risk of heart disease in women.

People with high levels of BPA in their urine were found to have an increased prevalence of cardiovascular disease, according to one recent study.

Then a research team from the University of Cincinnati exposed cells from rat or mouse hearts to BPA and/or estrogen. Low doses of BPA markedly increased the frequency of arrhythmic (heartbeat irregularities) events, and the presence of the primary estrogen hormone from humans only seemed to amplify this effect. If a fast heart rate affects the heart's ability to pump, it can lead to a heart attack. ("Bisphenol A exposure increases risk of abnormal heart rhythms in female rodents." *The Endocrine Society.* Press release. 10 Jun 2009.)

Less Stress, More Joy

Besides getting more sleep, you might get more giggles. Throughout the past 10-plus years, laughter has been suspected of being a helpful addition to medicine for pretty much whatever ails you. Laughing appears to increase blood flow and possibly expand arteries.

Earlier studies by Lee Berk, DrPH, MPH, a preventive care specialist at Loma Linda University, suggested that laughter seemed to increase the levels of two hormones: one that helps elevate mood (beta-endorphins), and one that helps optimize immunity (human growth hormone). At the same time, laughter may decrease three stress hormones, which, when chronically elevated, can be detrimental to the immune system: cortisol, epinephrine, and dopac.

Berk's new study looked specifically at the effect of laughter on 20 high-risk diabetic patients with hypertension and hyperlipidemia. One group received the standard medications for diabetes, hypertension, and hyperlipidemia, while the other group received the same medications, plus viewed self-selected humor for 30 minutes a day. After two months, the researchers noted that people in the laughter group had lower levels of various hormones and markers that suggested lower stress levels and lower levels of inflammation. There was a bonus, too—this group also showed an increase in good cholesterol. For example, after a year, HDL (good cholesterol) levels increased by 26 percent in the laughter group compared to 3 percent in the control group. C-reactive protein levels—a possible marker for inflammation—decreased by 66 percent in the laughter group compared with 26 percent in the control group.

More studies need to be done, of course, but it sure looks like there is something to be said for laughter and other positive emotions such as joy, hope, and optimism. (*American Physiological Society* Apr 2009.)

Music can make you happy as well. When is the last time you purposely played some joyful music and gave yourself a few moments of pleasure and inspiration? You might want to start making this a daily dalliance. A small study by the Preventive Cardiology program at the University of Maryland measured blood vessel function in 10 people while they listened to music that they said gave them a sense of joy. The researchers discovered that their blood vessels dilated by 26 percent. This is similar to the beneficial response in blood vessel function that occurs after aerobic exercise. Imagine how happy your blood vessels would be after a session of aerobic exercise where you listened to all sorts of music that you love and find inspirational!

The situation went quite the other way, though, when the volunteers listened to music that made them anxious—their blood vessels narrowed by 6 percent. In general, country music made most of the volunteers feel joyful, while heavy metal music made them feel anxious. Maybe it's a good thing the music we tend to like in our golden years, when we are most at risk for heart disease, is a departure from what we listened to as teenagers. (*American Heart Association* Nov 2008.)

Exercise Helps the Heart

Getting some exercise and being physically active is a beautiful thing for your body, mind, and spirit. Exercise can be a powerful stress reducer and a mood elevator for some people. That's a great start—and past studies have shown that when people exercise on a regular basis, they tend to feel better about their bodies regardless of weight loss.

Exercise helps prevent heart attacks by improving blood pressure and blood cholesterol levels and by discouraging inflammation in the body by changing levels of various blood chemicals and improving blood vessel function.

What happens to your heart disease risk when you aren't exercising? Physical inactivity alone was associated with a 44 percent greater rate of cardiovascular events, according to a recent study that followed more than 1,000 people with heart disease for about six years. (Whooley M. et al. *Journal of the American Medical Association* 300: (2008): 2379–2388.)

Does exercise help patients with heart failure?

Researchers at the Duke Clinical Research Institute studied the effects of exercise on men and women with a significant degree of heart failure. The most important thing they discovered was that exercise—hopping on a stationary bicycle or a treadmill for just 25 to 30 minutes most days—is not only safe, but also effective in lowering the risk of hospitalization or death for this group. Check with your doctor first before starting a new exercise program, especially exercise programs that involve weight training. ("Exercise is safe, improves outcomes for patients with heart failure." *Journal of the American Medical Association*. 8 Apr 2009)

Sources

"Heart Disease and Stroke Pevention: Addressing the Nation's Leading Killers." Centers for Disease Control and Prevention 17 Dec 2009.

New England Journal of Medicine 360 (2009): 1179–1190

Akesson A. *Archives of Internal Medicine* 167 (2007): 2122–2127.

American Stroke Association. News Release 2008.

Archives of Internal Medicine 167(2007): 1951–1957.

Whang W., et al. "Depression and Risk of Sudden Cardiac Death and Coronary Heart Disease in Women" and Chida Y., et al "The Association of Anger and Hostility with Future Coronary Heart Disease." *Journal of the American College of Cardiology.* 17 Mar 2009.

International Association of Dental Research General Session. Apr 2009 poster session.

"Smoke from cigarettes, cooking oil, wood, shift male cardiovascular system into overdrive." American Physiological Society. press release. 17 Apr 2009.

Spiegel, et al. "Brief Communication: Sleep Curtailment in Healthy Young Men Is Associated with Decreased Leptin Levels, Elevated Ghrelin Levels, and Increased Hunger and Appetite." *Annals of Internal Medicine* 141.11 (2004): 846–850.

"Sleep duration is associated with variations in levels of inflammatory markers in women." American Academy of Sleep Medicine. press release. 1 Jul 2009.

Journal of the American College of Cardiology. 52 (2008): 343–346.

"Bisphenol A exposure increases risk of abnormal heart rhythms in female rodents." The Endocrine Society. Press release. 10 Jun 2009.

122nd Annual Meeting of the American Physiological Society. Apr 2009.

Scientific Sessions. American Heart Association. New Orleans, LA. 8–12 Nov 2008.

Whooley M. et al. Journal of the American Medical Association 300: (2008): 2379–2388.

"Exercise is safe, improves outcomes for patients with heart failure." *Journal of the American Medical Association.* 8 Apr 2009.

Chapter 2

Know Your Numbers

If you have heart disease, there's a menagerie of numbers to know about—from blood pressure and blood sugar levels to blood triglycerides and high-density lipoprotein (HDL, known as "good" cholesterol) to blood markers that measure inflammation in the body. It's hard to keep up. It's best to know your numbers for all of these various risk factors so you can take active measures to reverse your risk—be it with diet and lifestyle changes or medication or both. Think of these numbers as your way of seeing progress. This chapter deals with all the numbers you need to know going forward.

Ninety percent of those with heart disease have at least one of the traditional risk factors. "If you look for them, you'll find them," says Dr. DeVane, "whether it's low levels of HDL, family history of heart disease, high blood pressure, etc."

Various tests help measure heart disease risk.

Blood Pressure

About 73 million U.S. adults are walking around with high blood pressure or hypertension. It's called "the silent killer" because there are absolutely no signs that you have it.

Blood pressure is the force of blood pushing against blood vessel walls. The measurement is two numbers: the top number (systolic blood pressure) measures the pressure when the heart beats; the bottom number (diastolic blood pressure) measures the pressure when the heart rests between beats.

High blood pressure is a consistent pressure of 140 systolic (or higher) and/or 90 diastolic (or higher). A healthy blood pressure is considered to be 120/80.

When you have high blood pressure, your heart has to pump harder and the arteries are under increased pressure, which can lead to injury of the artery walls, atherosclerosis, and coronary heart disease. High blood pressure is also associated with an increased risk of stroke and kidney damage.

Some people with high blood pressure are able to bring it down to normal levels by making changes in their lifestyle (diet and exercise), while others need to add medication to bring it down.

How to Improve Your Blood Pressure and Decrease Stroke Risk

Less than one-third of people with high blood pressure have it under control. When uncontrolled, it significantly increases the risk of heart attack and stroke. If you reduce your diastolic blood pressure by 2 mm Hg, it is estimated to result in a 15 percent reduction in risk of stroke and mini-strokes, and a 6 percent reduction in the risk of coronary heart disease.

Strokes happen when a blood vessel feeding the brain with blood gets clogged or bursts. If it's clogged, that part of the brain is no longer getting the oxygen and blood it needs to function. If the vessel bursts, causing an aneurism, that part of the brain is flooded with blood and can't function. When either of these happen, that part of the brain can no longer control certain parts of the body.

Major causes of stroke are high blood pressure, smoking, diabetes, high cholesterol, heart disease, and abnormal heart rhythm (atrial fibrillation).

Experts agree that maintaining a healthy weight, staying active, and not smoking are three of your best bets for managing blood pressure. For every 2.2 pounds lost, blood pressure falls about 1 point. The following are other ways to improve your numbers:

1. Follow the DASH diet. Dietary Approaches to Stop Hypertension (DASH) is an eating plan that has been proven to lower blood pressure in studies sponsored by the National Institutes of Health. The daily diet prescription calls for fruits and vegetables (eight to 10 servings a day), low-fat dairy foods (two to three servings a day), whole grains (six or more servings), limited added fat and oils (4-5 servings a week) nuts, seeds, and beans (two to three tablespoons), and no more than two 3-ounce servings of lean meat, poultry, or fish. This way of eating, which contributes less total fat and saturated fat than the typical American diet, resulted in lower blood pressure in people with high and normal blood pressures. But when the researchers added a reduction of sodium into the mix, it led to an even bigger decrease in blood pressure.

2. Limit sodium and salt. Trying to take in less than 1,500 mg of sodium a day is a formidable goal. If this seems like a big jump for you, start by staying below 2,400 mg a day. Then try staying below 2,400 mg a day.

3. Boost your intake of three key minerals: potassium, calcium, and magnesium. All three minerals are

found in foods featured in the DASH diet. Potassium helps prevent and control high blood pressure. It works as an electrolyte in the body, helping maintain a healthy balance of water in the blood and body tissues. Higher potassium items include: prunes and prune juice, potatoes with skin, orange juice, leafy green vegetables (spinach, Swiss chard, broccoli), bananas, tomatoes, avocados, cantaloupes, artichokes, and papayas. Other big potassium hitters are beans and peas, including lentils and lima beans; fish, shellfish, and clams; nuts (including almonds, brazil nuts, peanuts, soy nuts, and pistachios); and low-fat dairy and yogurt.

To get your calcium, choose low-fat dairy and dark leafy greens, which are helpful for other reasons as well. Magnesium is found in nuts and beans, certain leafy green vegetables (broccoli and spinach), and potatoes; smaller amounts are in whole grain foods, meats, seafood, and milk.

4. Use extra-virgin olive oil, and follow the Mediterranean diet when possible. Some new research is suggesting that there are blood pressure–lowering benefits to including extra-virgin olive oil in your daily diet. Perhaps this is thanks to its antioxidant content, which includes phenolic plant compounds (a grouping of phytochemicals). It might be possible to lower your systolic blood pressure about four points (if it's presently around 140), according to a new study. Systolic blood pressure dropped 3 percent when a group of healthy men who don't typically eat a Mediterranean type of diet started using extra-virgin olive oil in moderate amounts.

5. Drink hibiscus tea. When a group of people with the highest blood pressure at the start of the study drank three cups of hibiscus tea daily for six weeks, their

systolic blood pressure dropped by 13 points and their diastolic blood pressure dropped by 6.4 points. Although more research is needed, it is pretty amazing to think that making one change can have such big results.

6. Eat foods with soluble fiber. There is some evidence that foods rich in soluble fiber may help lower blood pressure. Soluble fiber-rich foods include oats, barley, vegetables (such as Brussels sprouts, sweet potatoes, cabbage, and carrots), citrus fruits, prunes, apricots, pears, apples, berries, peas, and beans.

7. Seach for soy nuts. Researchers from Beth Israel Deaconess Medical Center in Brookline, Massachusetts, found that a 1/2 cup of soy nuts may help women lower their blood pressure after menopause almost as well as taking some medication. This daily dose of soy nuts decreased systolic blood pressure by 10 percent and diastolic by 7 percent in women with high blood pressure. A larger study is needed to confirm these effects. Other research suggests there might be a favorable effect on blood pressure from soy in general and soy protein in particular.

Triglycerides

Triglycerides are unique in that we get them from the fat that is in the food we eat. The body digests the fat, and the triglycerides are absorbed through the intestinal wall, where they are packaged a little differently and then released into the bloodstream. At this point, they can be burned for energy or stored. The liver also packages triglycerides into large particles called very low-density lipoproteins (VLDLs). As VLDLs give up their fats to body cells, they become dense, cholesterol-rich particles, including LDLs that contribute to plaque in arteries.

Testing for triglycerides is more important than previously thought. High serum triglycerides are common in the United States, and that's a problem for several reasons. Many heart experts now see serum triglyceride levels as the third important risk factor for atherosclerosis (along with blood levels of HDL and LDL). It also appears that the more triglycerides in the bloodstream, the less HDL the body tends to make. That's what you call a double whammy for heart disease.

Triglycerides are traditionally measured via a blood test after an overnight fast, but this may be changing. It was the nonfasting triglyceride levels (measured two to four hours after eating) that were recently linked with cardiovascular problems, including heart attacks. One new study suggests that high triglyceride levels, measured after meals, may be making HDLs less protective by impairing their anti-inflammatory action.

For now, normal triglyceride levels are less than 150 mg/dL after fasting. Borderline high levels are 150 to 199. High levels are 200-plus. (*Atherosclerosis* 204:2 (2009): 424–428.)

How to Lower Triglycerides

Many people with high triglycerides are overweight, sedentary, and smoke. There are few well-established medication options for lowering triglycerides, so quitting smoking, losing weight, and getting daily exercise are vital. These three lifestyle changes, along with the dietary suggestions ahead, are your best bet for lowering triglycerides.

Lowering them has a lot to do with choosing smart carbs—the ones that come from whole plant foods—over processed and easily digested carbohydrate foods, and choosing smart fats over bad. Here are some specific things you can do to help lower serum triglycerides:

- Avoid a high-fat diet, since triglycerides come from the fat we eat.

- Replace saturated fat and trans fats with monounsaturated fats such as olive oil, canola oil, and most nuts.

- Reduce your intake of sugar and other processed carbohydrates such as white flour and white rice. Choose instead whole grain foods such as brown rice, whole grain breads and cereals, and whole grain pasta. In 10 out of 11 studies, lowering the glycemic index (more on this in Chapter 3) by at least 12 points reduced triglycerides by approximately 9 percent. (Miller, JC Brand. "The importance of glycemic index in diabetes." *American Journal of Clinical Nutrition* (Supplement) 59: 747S–752S.)

- If you drink alcohol, limit drinks to no more than one a day for women and two a day for men. Alcohol can dramatically boost triglyceride levels in some people.

- Maintain a healthy weight and exercise regularly—both help lower triglycerides. When you exercise, you burn triglycerides. (Check with your doctor before starting an exercise program.)

- Add omega-3 fatty acids from fish to your diet. Start by eating fish high in omega-3s such as salmon a couple times a week. Recent studies show this reduces serum triglycerides while increasing HDL cholesterol, especially if saturated and trans fats have been replaced.

- Add omega-3 fatty acids from plant foods to your diet. Start by switching to canola oil in your cooking. The other top plant sources of omega-3s are ground flaxseed, broccoli, cauliflower, cantaloupe, and red kidney beans. This may help reduce serum triglycerides along with total cholesterol and LDL cholesterol.

- Add soluble fiber. This may help lessen the potential increase in serum triglycerides and other blood fats seen in some people with diabetes who eat a high carbohydrate diet. You'll find soluble fiber in beans, oats and oat bran, barley, psyllium seed products, some fruits (apples, mango, plums, kiwi, pears, berries, citrus, and peaches), and some vegetables (artichokes, celery root, sweet potato, parsnip, turnip, acorn squash, potato with skin, brussels sprouts, cabbage, green peas, broccoli, carrots, green beans, cauliflower, asparagus, and beets).

Cholesterol

Total Cholesterol

We get cholesterol from the animal products we eat (especially egg yolk, higher fat meat, poultry skin, whole milk dairy, and shellfish), but our liver also makes about 1,000 mg of it a day. Plant foods do not contain any cholesterol.

Total cholesterol levels of 240 mg/dL or higher put you at high risk for heart disease. Total levels of 200 – 239 mg/dL are considered borderline high risk. Keep in mind, if your HDL number is high, the total cholesterol number might be a little higher because it includes the amount of HDL circulating as well.

HDL Cholesterol

About one-third to one-fourth of blood cholesterol is carried by HDL. It is called "good" cholesterol because a high HDL level seems to protect against heart attack, while low HDLs indicate a greater risk of heart attack and stroke. Experts describe HDLs as protective scavengers, removing LDL from the blood and the artery walls.

Strive for above 60 mg/dL of HDL. Low HDL is less than 40 mg/dL in men and less than 50 mg/dL in women.

Making HDLs Work for You

"Good" cholesterol is the unique blood lipid component that you want more of, because increasing the HDLs helps lower your heart disease risk. The final report from the National Cholesterol Education Program (NCEP) Expert Panel on the Detection, Evaluation, and Treatment of High Blood Cholesterol in Adults notes, "Although LDL receives primary attention for clinical management, growing evidence indicates that both VLDL (very low density lipoprotein cholesterol) and HDL play important roles in atherogenesis." Atherogenesis is the origination and formation of fatty deposits in arteries.

Researchers from Maastricht University in the Netherlands, who conducted an analysis of 60 controlled trials on dietary factors and blood lipids, now believe that the ratio of total cholesterol to HDL cholesterol is a more specific marker of coronary artery disease than the LDL blood cholesterol measurement. (Your total cholesterol value is divided by your HDL value from your lipid panel blood test.)

Boosting HDL just may be the next frontier in heart disease prevention. Dr. P. K. Shah, director of cardiology at Cedars-Sinai Medical Center in Los Angeles, believes that if the new drugs that increase levels of HDLs work, we could potentially reduce the number of heart attacks and strokes by 80 to 90 percent and save millions of lives.

Experts don't know for sure yet how HDL cholesterol helps reduce the risk of heart disease, but there are a few thoughts on this. The NCEP's report states that high levels of HDL appear to protect against the formation of fatty plaques in the artery walls (atherogenesis), according to studies with genetically modified animals. In vitro studies suggest that HDLs promote the removal of cholesterol from foam cells in atherosclerotic lesions. "Recent studies indicate that the antioxidant and anti-inflammatory properties of HDL also inhibit atherogenesis," the report notes.

(*Circulation* 106:25 (2002): 3143–421. *Journal of the American Medical Association* 285:19 (2001): 2486–97.)

The good news is we can boost our HDL levels through diet and lifestyle.

- Replace saturated fats with monounsaturated fats.

- Exercise 30 minutes or more a day.

- Don't smoke.

- Drink moderate amounts of alcohol. A few words about this. Consuming alcohol, especially with meals, appears to do two things to help reduce heart disease risk in humans. Dr. Byung-Hong Chung, PhD, conducted a study that provided evidence of alcohol-related effects that reduce cardiovascular disease risk. According to Chung, alcohol increases HDL cholesterol levels and enhances the movement of cholesterol deposits out of cells lining the arterial walls. Alcoholic drinks may be beneficial, but keep them to no more than one a day for women and no more than two a day for men.

- Lose weight if you are extremely overweight. Being overweight or obese is listed as one of eight causes for low HDL levels, according to the NCEP report. There could be several mechanisms at play here, but we do know that obesity tends to raise serum triglyceride levels, which consequently tend to lower HDLs.

LDL Cholesterol

Low-density lipoprotein (LDL) is the major cholesterol carrier in the blood. Together with other substances, it can form plaque deposited in artery walls. That's why it's called "bad" cholesterol. Here are the numbers to know:

- 160 mg/dL and above is considered very high and reflects an increased risk of heart disease.

- Achieving an LDL of below 100 mg/dL is now widely recommended for patients with two or more risk factors for heart disease and for those with diabetes but no other major heart disease risk factors.

- A target of LDL at or below 70 mg/dL is recommended for patients with established heart disease or with diabetes and additional risk factors for heart disease (such as high blood pressure, tobacco use, or family history of heart disease).

How to Lower Your LDLs

Almost 54 million women and just over 48 million men have total cholesterol levels higher than 200 mg/dL. That's more than 100 million people. If that doesn't scare you, this should: Most people who suffer a heart attack each year have only mildly elevated cholesterol levels. Cholesterol does not need to be shockingly high to contribute to heart disease. All those people could benefit from even a 10 to 20 percent reduction in their total cholesterol.

If we are going to study the way diet influences heart disease risk, we have to look at how what we eat raises or lowers LDLs. It has long been known that saturated fat raises LDL numbers, and the same foods that are high in saturated fat tend to contribute to dietary cholesterol. Recent clinical trials robustly show that LDL-lowering therapy reduces heart disease risk. The following are diet measures you can take to lower LDLs:

- Reduce your intake of saturated fat and eliminate trans fat altogether. Limit full-fat dairy products, higher-fat red meats, poultry skin, stick margarine, cookies, crackers, and fast-food french fries. A product's nutritional information should indicate that the saturated fat content is less than 7 percent of the total calories.

- Switch to smart fats (monounsaturated fat and omega-3s). They're found in fish, plant foods, nuts and seeds, olive and canola oil, and ground flaxseed. A recent study found that people who enjoyed 1.5 ounces of walnuts a day for four weeks had lower LDL levels. Walnuts contribute plant omega-3s plus assorted helpful phytonutrients.

- Reduce your intake of food cholesterol to less than 200 mg/dl.

- Consume 2 grams per day of plant stanols and sterols (phytosterols help decrease the absorption of cholesterol).

- Increase soluble fiber intake to 10–25 grams per day.

- Switch to whole grains (especially oats)—they help lower LDLs, and they may improve insulin sensitivity as well.

- Control your weight. Lose some if you're obese, and maintain weight loss.

- Increase your physical activity.

- Have some flaxseed. ("Executive Summary of the Third Report of the National Cholesterol Education Program Expert Panel on Detection, Evaluation, and Treatment of High Blood Cholesterol in Adults" *Journal of the American Medical Association.* 285:19 (2001)). Although some studies have shown no effect, several studies have shown that one to two tablespoons of ground flaxseed a day reduces the LDL levels in people with high blood lipids.

- Eat almonds. A recent study found that when almonds were used as snacks in the diets of people with elevated blood lipids, their coronary heart disease risk factors significantly reduced, probably due in part to the fiber and monounsaturated fat components of almonds. (Kendall, et al. "Dose response of almonds on coronary heart disease risk factors". *Circulation* 106:11 (2002): 1327–1332.)

- Eat a vegetarian diet that includes cholesterol-lowering foods. Soy milk, soy burgers, oats, almonds, and bean soup along with fruits and vegetables have all been found to lower cholesterol levels. They may lower lipid levels as much as some medications.

- Look for lignan-rich plant foods. The phytoestrogen grouping of lignans may help block the oxidation of LDL, which means fewer of them will be depositing in your arterial walls. You can find lignans in ground flaxseed, kidney beans, soybeans, lentils, navy beans, pinto beans, pears, plums, asparagus, beets, bell peppers, broccoli, carrots, cauliflower, leeks, onions, snow peas, squash, sweet potatoes, and turnips.

ApoB

ApoB is a molecule present in cholesterol particles that significantly contributes to the development of plaquing or hardening of the arteries. The thought is that ApoB is a more accurate measure of the total number of all artery-clogging particles and thus a better indicator of heart risk than total cholesterol or LDL cholesterol.

ApoB testing may be particularly helpful in heart patients who have lowered their LDL cholesterol to recommended levels, according to an expert statement from the American College of Cardiology. If ApoB levels are high, the panel concluded that patients might need more aggressive lifestyle interventions or larger doses of lipid-lowering statin drugs, even if their LDL levels are within normal range.

What do the numbers mean? Less than 90 is the target for high-risk patients without established heart disease. Less than 80 is the target for the highest-risk patients with heart disease or with diabetes and other cardiovascular risk factors.

High sensitivity C-reactive protein (hs CRP)

The liver makes this protein in response to infection, tissue injury, and inflammation, and it is thought to measure inflammation throughout the body. The test is not necessarily useful for people already diagnosed with heart disease or who are clearly at low risk for the disease, but it might be useful for people in the gray zone.

As for the numbers, a healthy level is less than 1 mg/L. If they fall between 1 and 3 mg/L, you have an intermediate risk. Above 3 mg/L is high risk. A test result above 10 mg/L suggests some other inflammation-related condition is present.

There are several ways you can encourage a decrease in levels of hs CRP. All of these help decrease the risk of heart disease in general:

- Quit smoking.
- Maintain or achieve a healthy weight.
- Get plenty of omega-3-rich foods from fish (salmon, albacore tuna, sardines) and plants (canola oil, ground flaxseed, walnuts).
- Adopt a Mediterranean-style diet based on fruits, vegetables, whole grains, nuts, and olive oil.
- Exercise almost every day.
- Get enough sleep.
- Reduce stress.

Heart Rate or Pulse Rate (for Postmenopausal Women)

Resting pulse rate (heart rate) was found to be a good predictor of heart attack risk in postmenopausal women, regardless of risk factors such as smoking, physical activity, and alcohol consumption. Researchers analyzed data from postmenopausal women with no history of heart problems. Those with the highest heart rates were much more likely to suffer a heart attack in an eight-year period than women with the lowest resting pulse rates. (Hsia J. et al. *British Medical Journal*. 338 (2009): b219)

What do the numbers mean? The highest resting heart rates are 76 beats per minute or higher. The lowest resting heart rates are 62 beats per minute or lower.

Sources

Atherosclerosis 204:2 (2009): 424–428.

Hsia J. et al. *British Medical Journal*. 338 (2009): b219

"Executive Summary of the Third Report of the National Cholesterol Education Program Expert Panel on Detection, Evaluation, and Treatment of High Blood Cholesterol in Adults" *Journal of the American Medican Association*. 285:19 (2001).

Kendall, et al. "Dose response of almonds on coronary heart disease risk factors." *Circulation* 106:11 (2002): 1327–1332.

Miller, Brand JC. "The importance of glycemic index in diabetes." *American Journal of Clinical Nutrition*(Supplement) 59: 747S–752S.

Circulation 106:25 (2002): 3143–421.

Journal of the American Medical Association 285:19 (2001): 2486–97.

"National Cholesterol Education Program (NCEP) Expert Panel on the Detection, Evaluation, and Treatment of High Blood Cholesterol in Adults." *Circulation*. 106: 25 (2002): 3143–421.

Arteriosclerosis, Thrombosis and Vascular Biology, Jul 2001.

Journal of the American College of Nutrition 18:3 (1999).

American Journal of Clinical Nutrition Jun 2001.

Nutrition and Cancer 39:2 (2001)

Cancer Epidemiology Biomarkers and Prevention. Sep 1997.

Environmental Nutrition Jun 2003.

ESHA Research Food Processor II nutrition analysis software, 2003.

Chapter 3

10 Steps You Can Take Today to Slow and Possibly Reverse Heart Disease

I'm about to throw some serious nutrition habits and changes at you. I know that even the most motivated nutrition-conscious people can't do all of these every single day. You can probably guess what some of these food steps are by now based on what I've said in the previous chapters. Whether we're talking about lowering blood lipids and blood pressure or protecting your heart and arteries from inflammation and atherosclerosis, the advice is the same. When you put it all together, it will make sense.

In general, you don't want to eat a diet high in saturated fat, trans fat, sodium, cholesterol, and extra calories (from sugary, high-fat foods). You do want to eat a diet with lots of smart carbs (fruits, vegetables, whole grains, beans) and smart fats (fish and plant foods rich in omega-3s and monounsaturated fat such as nuts, olive oil, canola oil, and ground flaxseed). A handful of nutrients have been linked to anti-inflammatory action (betaine, choline, fiber, vitamin D, vitamin K, and zinc), and their food sources basically lead us down this same dietary path.

The bottom line: Eat more whole foods and less processed foods, junk foods, and fast foods. Try to enjoy more whole grains, fish, dark green and cruciferous vegetables (broccoli, cauliflower, cabbage, brussel sprouts, bok choy, kale), a variety of fruits, nuts, and beans. When cooking and baking, try to use canola oil and olive oil in sensible amounts when possible. One of the most important dietary strategies is to decrease saturated fat and eliminate trans fat altogether. If you eat animal foods or products, gravitate toward the leanest meats, skinless poultry, and skim and reduced-fat dairy products (preferably fortified with vitamin D).

What about supplements?

The potentially beneficial supplements that you will want to discuss with your cardiologist include ground flaxseed (1 to 2 tablespoons a day), fish oil capsules, and plant sterol–fortified margarines. The American Heart Association recommends 1 gram of fish omega-3s (EPA plus DHA) per day for patients with coronary heart disease under a physician's care. Until more research is conducted, however, fish oil supplements should not be taken by patients with angina or those with an implantable cardioverter defibrillator, according to a review on the treatment of cardiovascular disease in the February 2008 issue of the Journal of the Dietetic Association.

The 10 Steps You Can Take Today to Slow and Possibly Reverse Heart Disease

Step 1: Eat Like a Mediterranean More Often

By learning the Mediterranean diet, you are adopting a way of eating that helps protect your heart. Researchers aren't certain which mechanisms are at play, but they suspect it could involve a reduction in oxidative stress, anti-inflammatory effects, improvement in how the artery walls function, and/or changing blood lipid levels.

The traditional Mediterranean-style of eating emphasizes:

- Extra-virgin olive oil as the primary source of fat.
- Whole grains (includes pasta, bread, and rice).
- Legumes or beans (chickpeas, lentils, fava beans).
- Fruits and vegetables (about nine servings a day).
- Nuts (about a handful a day).
- Fish (at least twice a week) that isn't fried, cooked with butter, or served with heavy sauces.
- Chicken (not deep fried, but roasted, grilled, or prepared with olive oil).
- Red wine (in moderation—no more than 5 ounces for women and 10 ounces for men daily, if the doctor approves).
- Herbs and spices as flavorings (instead of salt).

The diet de-emphasizes high-fat dairy such as whole or 2% milk, full-fat cheese and ice cream; red meat (very little red meat is eaten); and sausage, bacon, and other high-fat processed meats. Use of butter with bread and in baking is minimized along with the use of products made with hydrogenated or partially hydrogenated oils.

The Mediterranean diet may also help prevent type 2 diabetes. According to a Spanish study, those who followed a Mediterranean diet over a four-year period were less likely to develop type 2 diabetes, regardless of other factors such as family history of diabetes and physical activity. When the diet includes an ounce of nuts a day, it may improve the management of metabolic syndromes as well. (Martinez-Gonzalez, Miguel A. "Anatomy of health effects of Mediterranean diet: Greek EPIC prospective cohort study." *BMJ*. 338:b2337. 23 Jun 2009.)

In addition, people who closely followed the traditional Mediterranean diet had significant health improvements in several areas, according to an analysis of 12 international studies. They enjoyed a 20 percent drop in overall death rates, a 9 percent drop in death from cardiovascular disease, and a 13 percent drop in incidence of Parkinson's and Alzheimer's. (Cesari F. et al.,"Adherence to Mediterranean diet and health status: meta-analysis." *BMJ*. 337:a1344 11 Sep 2008. Mitrou, PN. *Archives of Internal Medicine* (2007))

However, there are two aspects to the Mediterranean diet that require caution. Be careful not to eat too much fat. Even the good kind of fat is high in calories (9 calories per gram) and, if eaten in excess, will contribute to weight gain and obesity. And be careful not to drink too much alcohol. Some people can't stop at one or two drinks. In that case, it would be better to eliminate alcohol from the diet completely.

Step 2: Strive to Stay Below 1,500 mg of Sodium Per Day

Admittedly, staying around or below 1,500 mg of sodium per day is going to be tough. One measly frozen entrée uses up half your daily sodium allotment; even the better ones have around 800 mg. Have a grilled chicken sandwich at a fast food chain, and there goes the other half (about 1,100 mg per sandwich).

It's going to be tough to work this food step, but it's doable. It will take some major shifts in food choices and kitchen habits. There are good reasons to keep at it.

A diet high in sodium increases the risk of having high blood pressure, which is a major cause of heart disease and stroke, the first and third leading causes of death in the United States. According to a new study by the Centers for Disease Control and Prevention (CDC), more than two out of three American adults are in population groups that should consume no more than 1,500 mg of sodium per day. These population groups include persons with high blood pressure, African Americans, or people age 40 and over. If you're not in one of these groups, then the maximum recommended daily amount gets bumped up to 2,300 mg a day.

Most Americans consume more than double the amount of sodium recommended. The average intake of sodium for Americans age 2 years and older was 3,400 milligrams per day in 2005 and 2006, according to the CDC. This amount is shocking enough, but it may even be an underestimation of our true intake because this figure comes from a national survey that did not include salt added at the table or during home cooking. The Center for Science in the Public Interest (CSPI) estimates that the actual average consumption of sodium is probably closer to 4,000 milligrams a day.

For those who need to stay below 1,500 mg of sodium a day, this should be a top priority starting yesterday. How do we stop the sodium surge? Most of the sodium we take in comes directly from processed and packaged foods and the food we buy at fast food chains and restaurants. So our first few tips address those:

- Know how much sodium is in a serving of a food product you are about to buy. Read the label. You'll be very surprised to see how many milligrams of sodium per serving there are in many products. Make a lower sodium choice—low-sodium chicken broth, frozen entrees, or bottled marinara—whenever you can.

- Watch out for super high sodium fast-food items. Some fast-food selections far exceed the 1,500 mg daily limit. The Bacon Ultimate Cheeseburger from Jack in the Box contains 2,040 mg. The Premium Crispy Chicken Club Sandwich adds 1,830 mg to the meal. Order the Deluxe Breakfast or Big Breakfast at McDonald's, and you've added 2,150 mg and 1,560 mg, respectively, to your sodium levels. Once a fast-food chain or restaurant (or food manufacturer) adds salt or another high sodium ingredient to the product, you can't get it out.

- Rediscover the art of home-style cooking. There are so many good reasons to cook at home instead of buying processed and packaged foods. You save money, add more powerful nutrients to your daily diet, use the ingredients you want, and control the amount of salt in the food by using lower sodium options, salt-free seasoning blends, and fresh herbs for flavor. Cooking at home is the best way to lower the sodium in your diet.

- Reduce the amount of salt called for in most recipes. Salt is usually added to recipes as a flavor enhancer, so the amount can often be cut in half or left out completely. In the case of yeast bread recipes, however, it's best to add the salt called for because it helps control the yeast activity. Keep in mind that for every teaspoon of salt you cut out of your recipe, you are reducing the total sodium by 2,360 milligrams.

- Keep the salt shaker out of reach. Some people are in the habit of automatically adding salt to their food before they have even tasted it. Shake that habit by keeping the salt shaker out of reach. You can replace the salt shaker with a pepper mill or salt-free seasoning blends like Mrs. Dash, which comes in many different fun flavors. For every time you don't use the salt shaker (which adds 1/4 teaspoon of salt), you are reducing your daily sodium by 590 mg.

- Eat less processed foods. The Food Standards Agency of the United Kingdom estimates that 75 percent of salt intake comes from processed food. So, it seems the easiest way to take in less sodium is to eat less processed foods. Some food companies are developing products with less sodium, so read the food labels. Only small amounts of sodium occur naturally in foods, so fill your meals with mostly natural, whole foods to help keep sodium levels down.

- Cut down on some condiments. Always dress your sandwiches and burgers yourself. That way, not only can you control the amount, you can use condiments such as the following, that are lower in calories, fat, and sodium:

- Balsamic vinegar, 2 teaspoons, contributes 14 calories, 0 grams fat, and 2 mg sodium
  - Mustard, 1 teaspoon, contributes 10 calories, 0 grams fat, and 100 mg sodium
  - Pickle relish, 1 tablespoon, contributes 21 calories, 0 grams fat, and 109 mg sodium
  - Horseradish, 2 teaspoons, contributes 4 calories, 0 grams fat, and 10 mg sodium
  - Lemon juice (from 1/2 lemon) contributes 8 calories, 0 grams fat, and 1 mg sodium.
- Feel free to load on all the lettuce, tomato, and onion your heart desires. Each of these adds 5 calories or less per serving and almost no sodium.
- Beware of dressings and sauces. If you think a little bit of dressing or sauce isn't going to add that much sodium to your meal, think again. Take a gander at some of the dressings offered at Jack In The Box. The Creamy Southwest Dressing packet has 1,060 mg sodium. The Bacon Ranch Dressing packet has 810 mg sodium. And the Asian Sesame Dressing packet has 780 mg sodium.

Step 3: Drink Wisely (Kick the Soda Habit)

What you choose to drink each day can help or harm your health and your heart. Are you drinking liquids that contribute calories without nutrients? These calories, which add up pretty quickly through the day, are more likely to be treated like "extra" calories by your body, leading to body weight gain. Recent studies suggest that when we drink our calories in beverage form, they don't seem to register to our stomach the way food calories do.

In other words, it's better to eat your carbohydrate calories than to drink them. Obesity experts agree that beverages are a major contributor to the alarming increase in obesity.

There are other options. We could drink beverages that help protect our health by contributing phytochemicals that have powerful antioxidant action in our body. This would be the case with green, white, and black tea.

But what is it about soda that makes it such a tough habit to break? Is it the bubbles from carbonated water? Is it the caffeine? Part of the reason it is so addicting is that these quick carbohydrate calories seem to stimulate cravings and further consumption of liquid and more food.

Americans should cut back on their intake of the two sweeteners used in regular soda—fructose (a major source in soda is high fructose corn syrup) and sugar (also known as sucrose). The calorie contribution from beverages represents 21 percent of the total daily calories for Americans over two years of age. Perhaps more shocking is that the proportion of calories consumed from sweetened soft drinks and fruit "drinks" tripled between 1977 and 2001.

But is simply switching to diet sodas the answer to kicking the soda habit? I suggest people try to choose diet sodas that use Splenda. Even though "less is better" when it comes to alternative sweeteners, these noncaloric sweeteners are better than gulping down the 10 teaspoons of sugar in a regular can of soda. If you're a big soda drinker, try to dial it down to one diet soda a day. Save it for the time of the day when you really feel like having one. For me, this tends to be in the afternoon.

Kicking the soda habit comes down to three steps: Make up your mind to give it up; gradually switch to diet sodas and other calorie-free options; and stock up on non-soda options, such as green tea (white tea and black tea), soy milk, skim milk, mineral water, coffee (decaf is best later in the day), and good old H2O with a slice of lemon or lime.

Notice I didn't list fruit juice? Fruit juice is a concentrated source of fructose and even one serving a day has been shown to increase the risk of diabetes. Basically it's better to eat the orange, apple, or grapes (with all the fiber and nutrients) than to drink the juice.

Step 4: Put Your Powerful Phytochemicals to Work

There are three phytochemical families that stand out as being helpful and protective against cardiovascular disease: polyphenols, plant sterols/stanols, and lignans. I've mentioned them already, but I want to dig deeper into these powerful phytochemicals.

Polyphenols

Polyphenols are nature's pharmaceuticals. They are found in plants in small quantities, and their job is to protect plant cells. There is reason to believe these same polyphenols can also help protect animal cells in much the same way. Admittedly, we have much to learn and more research to perform concerning polyphenols, but so far it seems that scientists may have hit the nutritional mother lode when they identified this huge class of phytochemicals.

Some scientists believe polyphenols may be one of the most powerful sources of bioactive components being investigated in the coming years. Bioactives are food components, other than those needed to meet basic nutritional needs, that are responsible for changes in health status. Even in small amounts, polyphenols appear to help combat inflammatory disease by controlling gene expression.

Polyphenols are thought to do more than this. They may help lower blood pressure, may reduce the tendency of platelets to stick together, may improve blood lipids levels, may discourage atherosclerosis and help make blood vessels more open and flexible (which improves blood flow), may help improve blood glucose regulation, and may contribute to weight control and weight loss by speeding up the metabolism and possibly encouraging the body to burn more fat.

The polyphenol family of phytochemicals is huge and includes several subgroups with several phytochemicals within them. In the list ahead, you'll notice that many of the same foods are listed under different phytochemicals. That's because each plant food represents a potpourri of phytochemicals. The subgroups, Bioflavonoids and Phenolic Acids, represent the major polyphenols that appear to have protective action against heart disease, inflammation, or arterial plaquing.

For example, animal studies suggest the polyphenols—catechins and epicatechin—help reduce total cholesterol, LDLs, and triglycerides, while increasing good cholesterol levels. And the flavonols are reported to be the most effective of the polyphenols at reducing the tendency of platelets to stick together. One of the flavonols—kaempferol—may help dilate blood vessels. We need them all, and we need them now. Here are five of the main Bioflavonoids/Flavonoids (a major classification of phytochemicals) and what foods you can find them in:

1. Anthocyanins: Food sources: berries, purple grapes, red wine, eggplant, black and green tea.

2. Catechins/tannins: Food sources: cocoa powder and dark chocolate; green and white tea; oolong, Earl Grey, Ceylon and darjeeling black teas; lentils and black-eyed peas; grapes.

3. Ellagic Acid: Food sources: raspberries, strawberries, pomegranate, apples, grapes, walnuts.

4. Hesperitin and Naringin: Food sources: citrus fruits, particularly the pulp.

5. Flavonols—Quercetin and its breakdown product—Rutin, and Kaempferol: Food sources: apples, pears, tea, cherries, grapes, strawberries, kale, tomatoes, potatoes, onions, leeks, broccoli, endive, chives, red cabbage, radishes, apricots, citrus fruits, rhubarb, parsley, buckwheat.

Plant Sterols

By decreasing total and LDL cholesterol levels, plant sterols help reduce the risk for cardiovascular disease in people with elevated cholesterol levels. Here's how it seems to work. Phytosterols have a chemical structure similar to cholesterol, and when they are present in the intestinal tract, they help decrease the absorption of cholesterol through the intestinal wall in two ways. Phytosterols inhibit the absorption of the dietary cholesterol from the food we eat, and the reabsorption of cholesterol from bile acids (which the body secretes as part of normal digestion). The liver then starts taking LDL cholesterol from the bloodstream to make new bile acids and LDL cholesterol levels decrease.

Plant sterols and stanols in amounts of 2 to 3 grams a day decrease total cholesterol and LDL cholesterol levels by as much as 15 percent. When people with normal cholesterol levels ate some food products with plant sterols added (margarine, low-fat yogurt, bakery products) for four weeks or longer, total cholesterol decreased 4 to 8.9 percent and LDL cholesterol decreased 6 to 14.7 percent, according to three different studies. The daily dose of plant sterols ranged from 1.6 to 3.2 grams a day, depending on the study.

Various food products have plant sterols added. But you can also find impressive amounts of plant sterols naturally in healthful plant foods such as whole grains, fruits, nuts, and vegetables because sterols are part of the cell membranes in plants.

Here is a sampling of foods that naturally contribute plant sterols:

- Avocado (1/2 of a small): 132 mg
- Soybeans, 1/2 cup: 45 mg
- Chickpeas, 1/2 cup: 35 mg
- Almonds, 1 ounce: 34 mg
- Olive oil, 1 tablespoon: 30 mg

If you get plenty of plant foods in your diet, you'll get even more plant sterols because there are small amounts in many of the foods we know and love—and it all adds up. You'll also find phytosterols in brussels sprouts, legumes (beans), rye bread, whole wheat (in the wheat bran and wheat germ), seeds (particularly sunflower and sesame seeds), nuts (almonds, cashews, macadamia, peanuts), and canola oil.

Just eating the heart-smart way (plentiful in nuts, beans, vegetables, fruits, and whole grains) will get you easily to a desirable amount of phytosterols—about 600 mg per day!

Here is a sampling of food products that contribute plant sterols:

Product	Serving Size	Grams of sterols/ stanols per serving
Margarine		
Take Control	1 tablespoon	1.7
Take Control Spread	1 tablespoon	1.7
Take Control Spread Light	1 tablespoon	1.7
Smart Balance Heart Right Light	1 tablespoon	1.7
Benecol Spread	1 tablespoon	.85
Benecol Light Spread	1 tablespoon	.85
Smart Balance OmegaPLUS Butter Spread	1 tablespoon	.45
Orange Juice		
Minute Maid Heart Wise Orange Juice	8 ounces	1.0
Chews		
Benecol Smart Chews	1 chew	.85
Granola Bars		
Nature Valley Heart Healthy Granola Bar	1 bar	.4

Lignans

Lignans are one of several phytochemicals that have a structure similar to estrogen and are called phytoestrogens. Lignans exhibit anti-inflammatory actions. One of the ways they do this is by blocking the pro-inflammatory actions of platelet activating factor (PAF). PAF is produced by white blood cells and the immune system cells. Lignans also have antioxidant properties and may help block the oxidation of LDL cholesterol particles, encouraging fewer of them to deposit in your arterial walls.

You can get lignans from various sources. Ground flaxseed is one of the most lignan-rich plant foods on the planet, and most days I add a tablespoon of ground flax to my diet. But there are other lignan-containing plant foods that you might know and love and want to add to some of your meals as well. They include kidney beans, soybeans, lentils, navy beans, pinto beans, pears, plums, asparagus, beets, bell peppers, broccoli, carrots, cauliflower, leeks, onions, snow peas, squash, sweet potatoes, and turnips.

Adding 1 tablespoon of ground flaxseed to your food every day is an inexpensive habit to start. Flaxseed contains a high concentration of plant omega-3 fatty acids (around 1.5 grams per tablespoon) and lignans, which have anti-inflammatory and antioxidant properties. Each tablespoon of ground flaxseed contributes almost 3 grams of fiber, a combination of soluble and insoluble fiber.

Step 5: Switch to Smart Fats

Avoiding greasy, rich, high-fat food is a no-brainer. But we can improve our health even further by making smart fat choices. The smart fats are monounsaturated fat, fish omega-3s, and plant omega-3s.

When eaten as part of a healthy diet, these smart fats actually benefit the body. Monounsaturated fats help reduce the risk of heart disease, especially if they are replacing saturated or trans fat. They reduce blood pressure and LDL cholesterol and may help increase HDL cholesterol. If a diet high in monounsaturated fat is combined with eating fewer carbohydrates, it can also improve insulin sensitivity.

Some high monounsaturated fat foods are olive oil, canola oil, peanut oil, hazelnut oil, almonds and almond oil (and some other nuts), and avocados.

Here are four fast ways to switch to smart fats:

- Eat fish at least a couple times a week (talk with your doctor about fish oil supplements).

- Use olive oil and canola oil in your cooking and baking whenever possible, instead of cooking fats high in saturated or trans fat or oils high in omega-6s (like safflower and corn oil). Buy products that use either of the two good oils.

- Enjoy nuts almost every day as a garnish on salads or entrees or as a snack instead of junk food.

- Work in a tablespoon of ground flaxseed almost every day by adding it to your smoothies, yogurt, soups, stews, or breakfast cereal, or substitute 1/2 cup of ground flaxseed for 1/2 cup of the flour when baking a batch of muffins or a loaf of bread.

Omega-3 fatty acids, especially from fish, may help decrease blood clotting, decrease abnormal heart rhythms, reduce triglycerides, and promote normal blood pressure. Plant omega-3s are also helpful, because your body can convert a small amount of the plant omega-3s into the fish omega-3s. Plus there is some evidence that plant omega-3s lower heart disease risk as well, through different actions than fish omega-3s.

Omega-3s seem to have anti-inflammatory action within body tissues, and some researchers suggest getting more omega-3s to reduce the risk of inflammatory diseases. More needs to be known about all of this, but the future certainly looks bright for both fish and plant omega-3s.

Good sources of fish omega-3s obviously include fish, but cold-water fish such as salmon, tuna, mackerel, trout, herring, and bluefish are especially good. Canned tuna also contributes some omega-3s. For a handful of user-friendly fish recipes, check out Chapter 4.

The top plant omega-3 foods include flaxseed, walnut oil, canola oil, soybean oil, and English walnuts. Other plant foods that contribute omega-3s are soybeans, tofu, pecans, broccoli, and other green leafy vegetables.

Omega-6s are found in grapeseed oil, corn oil, some formulations of safflower oil and sunflower oil, peanut oil, soybean oil, products that contain one of these oils (like mayonnaise), and meats that are fed with corn (like chicken). Omega-6s are known to lower heart disease risk by replacing saturated or trans fat in the diet, yet they aren't considered smart fats.

When we eat omega-6s in excessive amounts—which happens with the typical Western diet—they can do two things. They can spur the production of hormone-like substances called eicosanoids, which leads to inflammation and damaged blood vessels by promoting blood clots and constricted arteries. And they interfere with the body's conversion of plant omega-3s to the more powerful fish omega-3s.

Our bodies are able to convert small amounts of plant omegas into the fish omegas, but if we have a lower amount of omega-6 in our diet, we are able to convert even more plant omega-3s to the longer-chain fish omega-3s. This is because when our bodies metabolize the omega-6s in our diet, we use the same enzyme that the body needs to convert plant omega-3s to the longer-chain fish omegas.

The typical American consumes about 10 times more omega-6s than omega-3s. Some experts suggest a healthier ratio would be three times the omega-6s to omega-3s.

How much omega-3 do we need? The recommendation to eat about eight ounces (2 to 3 servings) a week of fish rich in omega-3s—such as salmon, mackerel, and sardines—leads to an average daily intake of 500 mg combined of EPA and DHA, which is associated with a lower risk of heart disease. For those with heart disease, the recommendation for 1,000 mg EPA and DHA would require doubling this fish consumption and may lead some to take fish oil supplements.

The American Heart Association's recommendations for omega-3s are:

- Patients without documented coronary heart disease: Eat a variety of (preferably oily) fish at least twice a week. Include oils and foods rich in plant omega-3s (flaxseed, canola, soybean oils, and walnuts).

- Patients with documented coronary heart disease: Consume about 1 gram EPA plus DHA per day, preferably from oily fish. EPA plus DHA supplements could be considered in consultation with a physician.

- Patients needing serum triglycerides lowered: 2 to 4 grams of EPA plus DHA per day provided as capsules under a physician's care.

A Handful of Nuts a Day Keeps Heart Disease Away

One of the most heart-smart food habits you could begin is having a handful of nuts almost every day. This is my snack du jour for the afternoon. It satisfies my afternoon hunger and seems to keep my energy level nice and balanced. More and more research continues to show the heart healthy benefits of nuts. Some years ago there were scores of almond studies, and now some of the other nuts are proving healthful as well.

In several recent studies, people were given around 1 ounce of walnuts per day for various periods of time (from six weeks to six-months). Walnuts decreased LDL cholesterol 10 to 12 percent and serum triglyceride levels decreased 17 to 18 percent in two of the studies. On top of all these other blood lipid benefits, HDL cholesterol levels increased by at least 9 percent in two of the studies.

I have found it really easy to boost my diet with walnuts or almonds. Here's what I do. I buy a big bag of the nuts at one of the warehouse stores, keep them in the freezer so they stay as fresh as possible, and then add them to all sorts of baking recipes, green salads, chicken and tuna salad, oatmeal, pancakes, muffins, cookies, and brownies.

Step 6: Make the Switch to Smart Carbs

The problem with many low-carb diets is that they aren't necessarily low in calories. These diets can be tough to maintain, too, because they limit variety.

Despite what you may think, a lower-fat, higher-carb diet can indeed help you lose weight and improve your health. The key is to be smart about your food choices. Instead of cutting out carbs, we should capitalize on high-carb good guys such as fruits, vegetables, whole grains, and legumes ("smart carbs" that deliver fiber, vitamins, minerals, and phytochemicals) and minimize refined carbohydrates (white flour, white rice, all types of sweeteners) and sweetened beverages.

Your Smart Carb Lineup

Eat beans in place of high saturated fat meats a few times a week. I call beans "protein pellets" because they are big on plant protein. A 1/2 cup serving comes with around 9 grams of protein—15 percent of the recommended intake for women. These perfect protein packages come with a healthy supply of complex carbohydrates (around 27 grams per half cup) and fiber (about 11 grams per half cup). Beans also contain phytochemicals called saponins, which may prevent cancer cells from multiplying by influencing genetic material in the cells. Soybeans and red kidney beans even add some plant omega-3s into the equation.

Eat your veggies and fruits.

Is it a coincidence that, as Americans have been getting fatter throughout the last 10 years, fruit and vegetable consumption nationwide has declined nearly 14 percent?

Fruits and vegetables are traditionally high in nutrients and fiber and low in calories. A cup of steamed broccoli contains 44 calories and 4.7 grams of fiber. A large apple contains 125 calories and 4.2 grams of fiber.

There is overwhelming scientific evidence that fruits and vegetables provide vitamins, minerals, phytochemicals, antioxidants, and other substances that have synergy with each other and protect against a variety of chronic diseases, including cancer, coronary heart disease, cataracts, and a number of inflammatory diseases.

Many nutrition experts would argue five servings a day is the bare minimum. And yet, for many people, it's work to eat that many servings. How can we squeeze more fruits and vegetables into our diet?

Keep fruit out where you can see it, which may entice you to grab some for a snack. Or cut some up into a fruit salad, which may be more appealing. If you're just not interested in eating fruits and vegetables, add them to the foods you are interested in. Put fruit in yogurt, oatmeal, pancakes, french toast, or cottage cheese, and add vegetables to chili, stew, casseroles, pastas, pasta salad, and omelets. If you're eating out, ask for a side of fruit or vegetables as a substitute for the hash browns or french fries. If you're the kind of person who tends to let fruits and veggies go bad, keep bags of frozen fruits and vegetables in your freezer. If cost is a factor, buy whatever is in season, which is usually priced better, and look for specials.

Embrace the "brown" and switch to whole grains

When you think "whole grains," you might think the health benefits mostly have to do with the fiber, but it's actually much more than that. Whole grains are rich in an assortment of vitamins, minerals, and phytochemical compounds that alone or in combination are likely to have significant health benefits that go beyond the fiber. Whole grains may provide many health benefits, including protection from cardiovascular disease, ischemic stroke, diabetes, insulin insensitivity and resistance, obesity, premature death, and certain cancers.

Nine common whole grains you might find in your supermarket are brown rice, oats, whole wheat flour, rye flour, barley, buckwheat, bulgur (steamed and dried cracked wheat), millet, and quinoa.

What Are the "Bad" Carbs?

The "bad" carbs are the processed or refined grains and all things sugar. The average adult takes in about 20 teaspoons of added sugar every day, according to the USDA's recent nationwide food consumption survey. That's about 320 calories, which can quickly end up as extra pounds. Added sugars (caloric sweeteners) are sugars and syrups that are added to foods at the table or during processing or preparation, such as high fructose corn syrup in sweetened beverages and baked products. Experts are still investigating the extent to which the body might metabolically handle natural sugars (in dairy products and fruit) differently from added sweeteners. My guess is the added sugars have a tendency to stimulate hunger and body fat deposits in genetically susceptible people.

We do know for sure that added sugars tend to supply calories with few or no nutrients, and that's what puts "added sugars" on their way to being considered a bad carb.

In an effort to jump on the low-fat diet bandwagon, many Americans have been eating more fat-free and low-fat products. But what they don't know is that in many of these products, sugar is being substituted for fat, so we've really been trading fat for sugar and getting nowhere fast.

The USDA recommends that we get no more than 6 to 10 percent of our total calories from added sugar—that's about 9 teaspoons a day for most of us, just under the amount in one soda.

Double Your Fiber for Your Heart

Although the average American gets about 14 to 15 grams of fiber a day, most health recommendations strongly suggest getting double this amount. The Institute of Medicine, for example, recommends getting 14 grams of fiber for every 1,000 calories you need, or about 28 grams of fiber for the typical 2,000 calorie diet.

High-fiber diets are linked to a few specific health benefits that come in handy if you are trying to slow or reverse heart disease: lower LDL and total cholesterol, lower risk of being overweight, lower risk of higher waist to hip ratios, lower blood pressures, and lower triglyceride levels.

It's not just about the fiber, though. There is synergy in many of the plant foods that contribute fiber. Synergy is when components work together for maximum health benefit. So this is really about eating high-fiber foods such as whole grains, fruits, vegetables, beans and legumes, and nuts and seeds.

According to a grouped analysis of 10 different studies, you can anticipate a 12 percent reduction in coronary events and a 19 percent reduction in coronary deaths for every 10 gram increase in daily fiber intake.

The Heart Smart Fiber—Viscous or Soluble Fiber

Soluble fiber (viscous or gelatinous) works the hardest at lowering total and LDL cholesterol. It does this by interfering with bile acid absorption from the lower end of the small intestines, which means less bile acid is getting reabsorbed and recycled. This causes more LDL cholesterol to be removed from the blood and converted into new bile acids to replace the bile acids lost in the stool. There is even evidence that the presence of some viscous fibers in the intestines may decrease cholesterol synthesis, so you're beating cholesterol coming and going, so to speak.

Your best food sources of soluble fiber are oats and oat bran, barley, beans, psyllium seed products, apples, bananas, citrus fruits, carrots, green beans, and ground flaxseed. The following are the top 30 viscous foods:

Food	Soluble Fiber (g)	Total Fiber (g)	Calories	Protein
Passion fruit, purple, 1 cup	12.3	25	229	5
Guava, fresh, 1 cup	4.5	9	112	4
Navy beans, cooked, 1/2 cup	2.8	9.5	27	8
Refried beans, fat-free, 1/2 cup	2.5	6	110	7
Cranberry beans, cooked, 1/2 cup	3.4	9	120	8
Cheerios cereal, 1 1/2 cups	2.9	4.5	165	5
Kidney beans, red, cooked, 1/2 cup	2.7	7	112	8
French beans, cooked 1/2 cup	2.6	8	114	6
Split green peas, cooked, 1/2 cup	2.5	8	116	8
Asian pears, fresh, 1	2.4	4	51	1
Life cereal, plain, 1 1/2 cups	2.3	4	239	6
Rye crispbread crackers, 2 ounces	2.1	9	207	5

Pinto beans, canned, 1/2 cup	2.1	6	103	6
Black beans, canned, 1/2 cup	2.1	8	113	8
Orange, fresh, medium, 1	2.1	3	62	1
Pink grapefruit, fresh, 1	2.1	3	91	1
Parsnips, fresh slices, 1 cup	2	7	100	2
Oats, rolled old-fashioned, 1/2 cup	2	4	150	5
Mung beans, fresh, 1/4 cup	2	9	179	12
Savoy cabbage, cooked, 1 cup	2	4	35	3
Baby lima beans, cooked, 1/2 cup	1.9	7	115	7
Brussels sprouts, cooked, 1 cup	1.9	4	56	4
Persimmon, Japanese, fresh, 1	1.7	6	118	1
Mango slices, 1 cup	1.7	3	107	1
Kiwifruit, 2	1.7	5	93	2
Blackberries, 1 cup	1.7	7	90	2
White beans, cooked, 1/2 cup	1.6	6	124	9

Pumpernickel bread, 2 slices	1.6	3	130	5
Oat bran, 1/4 cup	1.5	5	58	4
Flaxseed, ground, 2 Tbsp.	1.5	4	86	3

Step 7: Ban Trans Fat and Cut Back on Saturated Fat

Saturated fat receives the "bad fat" label because it raises LDL cholesterol and total cholesterol, which increases the risk of heart disease and stroke. Saturated fat can only be reduced or limited, because it is found in nature and would be virtually impossible to eliminate completely.

Trans fats, however, are mostly man-made and can be nearly eliminated. Trans fats do occur naturally in low levels in meat and dairy products, but most of the trans fats in the American diet are formed during partial hydrogenation of vegetable oils. They carry the title of "really bad fat."

Partial hydrogenation was patented in 1903. Its use in manufacturing food products increased in the 1950s, extending to margarines in the 1970s. It wasn't until the 1990s that studies started to identify trans fat as a health catastrophe. Trans fats lower HDL cholesterol and raise blood levels of LDL cholesterol, even at low levels of food intake. Trans fats also elevate a type of circulating cholesterol (lipoprotein (a) which is LDL cholesterol bound to the protein apolipoprotein (a)), which is thought to help inflame and stiffen the arteries. Experts estimate that a 2 percent increase in calorie intake from trans fat may increase the risk for a coronary event by up to 23 percent.

Baked goods, by the way, are the largest dietary source of trans fat.

As we move forward to phase out trans fats and the use of partially hydrogenated oil, we need to make sure that food suppliers aren't replacing them with saturated fats, like the tropical oils (palm, palm kernel, coconut) or animal fats, because that's what's available and affordable. I've noticed that as some of the fast-food chains have eliminated the trans fat in various items, the grams of saturated fat have increased simultaneously.

Can you imagine eating a serving of a particular food product only to find out later you just ate more than double the recommended intake of trans fats? That could easily happen because there are still plenty of products out there with 4 or more grams of trans fat per serving. The American Heart Association advises Americans to consume no more than 2 grams of trans fat per day.

The CSPI did its own survey in the spring of 2007 and found 45 products with at least twice (and in some cases three and four times) the maximum amount of trans fat recommended per day in just one serving of the product. Here are a few of the standouts:

Product	Trans fat (grams per serving)
Pepperidge Farm Pot Pie (Creamy Alfredo Chicken and Broccoli)	11
Tastykake Glazed Honey Bun	8
Edwards (Schwan) Chocolate Cheesecake	6
Wal-Mart Bakery Apple Fritters	6
Wal-Mart Bakery Iced or Glazed Honey Buns	6
Celeste Pizza for 1 (Original)	5
Keebler Club and Cheddar Sandwich Crackers	5
Keebler Vienna Fingers Cookies	5
Krispy Kreme Mini Crullers Doughnuts	5

Marie Callender's Razzleberry Pie	5
Pepperidge Farm Puff Pastry Shells	5
Pepperidge Farm Apple Turnovers	5
Pop Secret Homestyle Popcorn	5

How to Cut Back on Saturated Fat

There's no better way to cut back on saturated fat than by reducing the top three sources of saturated fat in the American diet: cheese, beef, milk. Just doing this hits more than 35 percent of the saturated fat we typically consume. Here are the eight main sources of saturated fat.

1. Cheese: Switch to reduced-fat cheese whenever possible, and use less regular fat cheese.

2. Beef: Choose leaner cuts, trim off any fat you can see, add small amounts of smart fats when preparing them, stick to sensible serving sizes, and eat red meat less often.

3. Milk: Switch to skim or 1 percent milk or fat-free half-and-half for cooking certain recipes.

4. Oils and other fats: Avoid deep-frying or cooking with large amounts of fat, switch to canola and olive oil in your recipes when possible, and use sensible amounts, even when using these smart fats.

5. Cakes/cookies/quick breads/doughnuts: Eat the higher fat bakery items less often, and when you do enjoy them, keep your serving size small. Make these items at home, and switch to canola oil or light margarine with plant sterols when you can.

6. Margarine: Buy a margarine that has the least amount of saturated and trans fat, but tastes good so you will be satisfied with smaller servings.

7. Butter: Buy whipped butter if you still want to
    use butter, and use less than the recipe calls for.
    Whipped butter contains 7 grams of total fat and
    5 grams of saturated fat per tablespoon, compared
    to stick butter, which has 11.5 grams total fat and
    7 grams of saturated fat. Switch to canola or olive
    oil or light margarines when you can.

8. Ice cream/sherbet/frozen yogurt: Stick to a 1/2-
    cup serving, and find some light ice creams and
    frozen yogurts that you truly enjoy.

Step 8: Avoid High AGE Foods

There is new wisdom in avoiding high-fat meats, deep-fried
foods, and fast foods. This time, it's all about avoiding Advanced
Glycoxidation End Products (AGEs), which are the new nutritional bad boys—found in these fatty foods—because they are
pro-inflammatory and pro-oxidant compounds.

In his research, Jaime Uribarri, MD, Nephrologist and professor
of Medicine at the Mount Sinai School of Medicine in New York, has
seen evidence of AGEs contributing to the impairment and injury of
the cells lining our blood vessels, lymphatic vessels, and heart. And
it doesn't take long for this dangerous action to take place—damage can begin just one to two hours after a high AGE meal. Most
Americans are constantly ingesting meals and snacks with a high
AGE content. The more AGEs circulate in our bodies, the more
problems they cause. Animal research has shown that a reduction
in circulating AGEs led to a reduction in the progression of two
key diseases: atherosclerosis and diabetes.

We need to start eating the low-AGE way. The good news is,
this way of eating goes nicely with all the other steps you've read
about in this chapter.

Eight Things You Need to Know About Eating the Low-AGE Way

If you want to start eating the low AGE way and reduce unwanted inflammation and oxidation in your body, here are eight things you need to know:

1. High heat cooking and dry heat cooking promote the formation of AGEs via glycoxidation and lipoxidation.

2. Changing your cooking methods, like stewing instead of frying chicken, can cut your AGE intake by more than 50 percent.

3. Using a marinade with an acid ingredient like lemon or vinegar will lower the AGEs in grilled meat.

4. Foods rich in both fat and protein and cooked at high heat and dry heat (grilling, frying, broiling) tend to have the highest amounts of AGE (possibly from high levels of free radicals being released during the oxidation of certain fats).

5. High AGE sources include full-fat cheeses, higher fat meats, and highly processed foods. Those were on our list to limit anyway!

6. Several food-processing techniques promote glycoxidation. Commercially prepared breakfast foods and snacks (like frozen waffles and Rice Krispies) seem to have significant amounts of AGE.

7. Some low-AGE protein sources include fish, skinless chicken breast, and low-fat and nonfat dairy products.

8. Low-fat, carbohydrate-rich foods, such as whole grains, fruits, and vegetables, tend to be relatively low in AGEs.

Results In a Month!

According to Uribarri, there will be health benefits from a low-AGE diet starting in two to four weeks, and these changes have been reported in research already. The ideal amount of change and further health benefits for the body, however, will come to fruition in a slightly longer period of time (approximately four months).

Reducing circulating AGE levels results in similar reductions in circulating CRP (C-reactive protein), a marker of inflammation in the body. A low AGE diet will also likely show beneficial changes related to diabetes and prediabetes. "I do believe that over the long-term, a low AGE diet also makes you lose weight when maintaining the same calorie intake," adds Uribarri.

Expect improvements in risk factors for diabetes and cardiovascular disease, with the bonus of weight loss or easier weight maintenance over time.

Step 9: Lose Weight Without Dieting

I won't belabor this point because we've all heard it before: Being obese increases your risk of all sorts of chronic diseases, including heart disease and stroke, in part by promoting inflammation in the body. Obesity more than doubles the risk for heart failure, according to new estimates. Overweight people are more likely to have heart disease "events" including heart attacks, even if their blood pressure and cholesterol are under control, according to the Centre for Prevention and Health Services Research in the Netherlands, which reviewed 21 studies on the subject.

The Dutch researchers found that, after adjusting for cholesterol and blood pressure, people who were overweight but not obese were 17 percent more likely to have a heart disease "event" compared to people with normal body mass indexes. The number increased to 49 percent more likely for people in the obese category. (*Archives of Internal Medicine* (2007): 1720–1728)

You've heard of apple and pear body shapes. Well, it's the apple shape—with the extra weight mostly being stored around the waist—that is most associated with heart disease and other diseases like metabolic syndrome and type 2 diabetes. This abdominal fat seems to be more biologically active, potentially secreting inflammatory proteins that contribute to atherosclerosis plaque. The bigger your waist, the higher your risk of developing heart failure—a condition where the heart isn't pumping enough blood out, and fluid and blood back up into the lungs and/or pool in the feet and legs.

In adults at the lower end of the "overweight" range in body mass index, an increase in waist circumference of 10 centimeters was associated with a 15 percent higher risk of heart failure for women and 16 percent higher for men. (*Circulation* online (2009)

Putting a Number to Your Waist

Measure your natural waist circumference (just above the navel) with a tape measure. If your body mass index (BMI) is 25 kg/m2 or greater (which is most of us), your goal for waist circumference, according to the American Heart Association, is less than 40 inches for men, and less than 35 inches for women.

What's the best way to bust belly fat? Exercise, exercise, exercise—plus I suggest limiting alcohol. Being obese makes it difficult to exercise, but exercising is crucial to keeping our hearts and bodies fit and healthy. Kinesiologists reported improvements in insulin sensitivity, less fat in the liver, and less inflammation in belly fat when obese mice engaged in moderate amounts of exercise, even without a change in diet. The mice's "moderate" exercise regimen was equivalent to humans walking 30 to 45 minutes a day five days a week. (University of Illinois at Urbana-Champaign. Press Release. 23 Apr 2009)

Slow-but-sure weight loss is likely to trim some of those waist inches off. That's often the first place our bodies put extra body fat, and that's where it will eventually come off.

Trim Extra Calories

No one particular weight-loss plan or program is more successful than another.

The only way to lose weight is to consume less calories than your body needs. No magic ingredients or food combinations will change this metabolic fact.

Your best bet is to eat when you are hungry and stop when you are comfortable, eat healthful whole foods you truly enjoy, and engage in regular exercise that you enjoy as well.

One of the best ways to trim extra calories is to avoid sweetened beverages such as soda, juice drinks, and bottled tea. Liquid calories aren't as satisfying as calories from food, and they can lead to consuming even more calories.

Is your eating environment helping or hurting? Does it encourage you to overeat or eat out of emotion? Stress and existing eating habits make it doubly difficult to stay on track and eat health-promoting foods while limiting health-damaging foods.

Be more attentive about the whole eating experience. When eating, be totally aware and in total enjoyment of your meals. When we eat in a distracted or hurried state, the food we just ate tends not to register well with our brain. Some experts recommend a pre-meal meditation to get centered before eating, but you can just take a couple of minutes to say a prayer or get to a quiet, more relaxed state.

What if you started focusing on happiness and health? Eat and exercise for the health of it, and let the pounds fall where they may. Let your body find its happy place by eating mostly healthy foods in healthy amounts and exercising on a regular basis—hopefully doing activities you enjoy. Just doing this will likely change the way you feel about your body. Get off the roller coaster of gaining and losing weight by making permanent changes in your lifestyle. The weight loss will be slower, but it's more likely to stay off this way.

The solution isn't weighing yourself every day, following a restrictive food plan that you can't do forever, or losing a certain number of pounds. The answer is living a healthy lifestyle. For most of you, doing this will naturally shed some of those extra pounds and, more importanly, will help your heart at the same time.

Step 10: The Heart Smart Journal

What if just by making one change in your habits you could double your weight loss? It may sound too good to be true, but many experts say that the simple act of keeping a food diary can encourage you to eat fewer calories and lose weight.

I admit the idea of writing down what you eat, how much, and other things (like your level of hunger on a scale of 1 to 10) might feel like a punishment and might put you in a "dieting and deprivation" frame of mind. But if you approach it more positively—like a tool to help raise your awareness about some of your food behaviors, and a way to improve your heart disease risk factors and increase your weight-loss success—it's worth a try, don't you think?

Several studies have shown that people who keep food journals are more likely to be successful in losing weight and keeping it off. In fact, a researcher from a recent study says that people who keep a food diary six days a week lost about twice as much weight as those who kept food records one day a week or less. For the six-month study, published in the *American Journal of Preventive Medicine*, dieters kept food diaries, attended weekly group support meetings, and were encouraged to eat a healthy diet and be active.

How does writing down what you eat and drink in a food journal work? For one thing, keeping a food diary instantly increases your awareness of what, how much, when, and why you are eating. This helps you cut down on mindless munching. Food diaries also help people identify areas where they can make changes that will help them with some of their heart disease risk factors and losing weight. The diaries can unveil patterns of overeating. They reveal triggers to avoid, such as when someone doesn't eat enough throughout the day and then overeats at night, or when someone tends to overeat when drinking alcohol.

For some people, the very fact that they have to record every bite helps deter overeating. People often find themselves reconsidering eating something because they don't want to write it down.

Eight Tips for Making the Heart Smart Journal Work for You

1. Know your reasons. If you know what you hope to gain from your food diary, you can make sure you're recording the type of information that will help you in that area. Megrette Fletcher (MeD, RD) advises people to be clear about their intent, whether it's to become aware of hidden food triggers, notice problematic eating patterns, or just make sure they're eating a healthy diet.

2. Choose your format. The basic elements dietitians often recommend for their clients are: time, food, amount/portion size, and degree of hunger. I've added the question, "How hungry am I?" in the Heart Smart Journal. You would write a number between 1 and 10 to represent the degree of hunger you have physically, with "1" being not hungry at all and "10" being ravenous.

    Some clinicians suggest including the location of the meal, because these details may provide insight into emotional triggers for eating habits, as well as times of day and places where healthy and unhealthy foods are most likely to be eaten.

    If you're trying to understand how your emotions relate to your food choices, you might also ask yourself, "What were my emotions before, during, and after the meal or snack?"

Keeping track of carbs, fat, and fiber grams will be helpful for people with diabetes and other medical conditions. If you have type 2 diabetes, you might find, for example, that meals high in carbohydrates or meals high in saturated fat may cause your blood sugar to soar. Or you might discover that your blood sugar levels improve when your meal or snack contains a certain amount of fiber or smart fat.

3. Decide how often to update. You can fill out your food journal as you go through your day, or set some time aside at the end of the day to update it. But experts say your record will be more accurate if you do it right after eating. They also say it's important to record everything—even if that seems painful.

   It can be tempting to avoid recording an unplanned indulgent dessert or binge episode, but this is the most important time to record. Something to watch out for: As time goes on, people tend to become more lax about how often they update their food journal and go longer after eating or drinking before logging the information.

4. Decide how detailed you want to be. If you just can't bring yourself to fill out the Heart Smart Journal form each day, that's okay. Just writing a minimum amount of information in your food journal will increase your awareness. People often believe that if they do not keep a "perfect" food log with every detail, they have failed. But keep in mind that every attempt you make at recording gets you a step closer to paying attention to your food choices and habits.

5. Be accurate about portion sizes. If you're just trying to get a general idea of what, when, and why you are eating, this tip may not apply to you. But if you want to get a precise picture of your intake (possibly so

a dietitian can do some quick calculations with it), make sure the amounts you record in your journal are as accurate as possible. Measuring out your portions in the beginning can help give you a picture of what certain amounts of food really look like. But if measuring food puts you in a dieting/deprivation mindset, you might want to skip the measuring and make your best guess.

6. Include the "extras" that add up. The more thorough you are when recording what you eat—that handful of M&Ms at the office, the mayo on your sandwich, the sauce on your entrée—the more ways you'll find to cut those extra calories. When you look back over your food diary records, look for those nibbles and bites that can really add up. Did you know that 150 extra calories in a day (one alcoholic drink or a slather of spread on your sandwich) could result in a 15- to 18-pound weight gain in one year?

7. Be aware of common obstacles. Are you embarrassed or ashamed about your eating? Do you have a sense of hopelessness, feeling that it won't help to fill out a food journal or that weight loss is impossible for you? Does it seem too inconvenient to write down what you eat and drink? Do you feel bad when you "slip up"? These are the four most common obstacles to keeping a food journal. What's the cure? All of these obstacles can be overcome by remembering the usefulness of the journal, not trying to be perfect, acknowledging that slips will happen, and staying motivated to use tools that promote health and well-being.

8. Review your information. Food journals are most helpful when you look back and review what you wrote. You can do this on your own or with a therapist or a dietitian who can help point out patterns that are keeping you from improving your health and suggest

alternatives to try. Just the process of writing things down is a big step toward awareness and understanding when and why you eat. Just asking the question, "How hungry am I?" reminds you to check in with your physical hunger. Review what you wrote, but don't make this an opportunity to bash yourself or feel failure. It's a process, and it's important to keep a positive attitude. I call it "journaling without judgment."

Sources

"Americans Consume Too Much Salt." *Center for Disease Control and Prevention.* Press Release. 26 Mar 2009.

Beasley, J. *Journal of the American Dietetic Association* 107:5 (2007): 739.

Burke L.E., *Contemporary Clinical Trials* 29:2 (2008): 182–193.

Catenacci, Victoria, MD, assistant professor of medicine, University of Colorado at Denver Health Sciences Center. Interview.

Cesari F. et al. "Adherence to Mediterranean diet and health status: meta-analysis". *BMJ.* 337:a1344 11 Sep 2008.

Cronin, Jeff. Director of Communications for the Center for Science in the Public Interest

Delinsky, Sherrie S., PhD, licensed staff psychologist, department of psychiatry, Massachusetts General Hospital. Interview.

Flynn, F.J. and D.R. Ames. *Journal of Applied Psychology* 91:2(2006): 272–281.

Gorman, Kim, MS, RD, director, Weight Management Program, University of Colorado, Denver. Interview.

Hawkins, Kerri Anne, MS, RD, dietitian, Obesity Consultation Center, Tufts Medical Center. Interview.

Hollis, J.F. *American Journal of Preventive Medicine* 35:2 (2008): 118–126.

Helsel, D. *Journal of the American Dietetic Association* 106:8 (2006): A46.

———. *Journal of the American Dietetic Association* 107:10 (2007): 1807–1810.

"Martinez-Gonzalez, Miguel A."Anatomy of health effects of Mediterranean diet: Greek EPIC prospective cohort study." *BMJ*. 338:b2337. 23 Jun 2009.

Megrette, Fletcher, MEd, RD, CDE, executive director, Center for Mindful Eating; co-author, Discover Mindful Eating. Interview.

Mitrou, PN. *Archives of Internal Medicine* (2007)

Puhl, Rebecca, PhD, director of research, Rudd Center for Food Policy and Obesity, Yale University. Interview.

Uribarri, Jaime, MD, Nephrologist and Professor of Medicine at the Mount Sinai School of Medicine in New York. Interview.

The Heart Smart Journal

Day___ Exercise_____ Medications_____

Meal #1 Time_____ Location_____

How hungry am I?

What are my emotions before this meal?

Food/beverage Amount Calories Sodium Sat. Fat Trans. Fat

How do I feel physically and emotionally after this meal?

Meal #2 Time_____ Location_____

How hungry am I?

What are my emotions before this meal?

Food/beverage Amount Calories Sodium Sat. Fat Trans. Fat

How do I feel physically and emotionally after this meal?

Meal #3 Time_____ Location_____

How hungry am I?

What are my emotions before this meal?

Food/beverage Amount Calories Sodium Sat. Fat Trans. Fat

How do I feel physically and emotionally after this meal?

Meal #4 Time_____ Location_____

How hungry am I?

What are my emotions before this meal?

Food/beverage   Amount   Calories   Sodium   Sat. Fat   Trans. Fat

How do I feel physically and emotionally after this meal?

Chapter 4

Heart Smart Versions of Your Favorite Recipes

We all have our favorite foods—those we love and look forward to eating, such as lasagna, hamburgers, and enchiladas. And let's face it, we are more likely to embrace heart-smart eating for years to come if we are able to still eat the foods we love. With a few tricks up your sleeve, this can be done most of the time. I've been lightening recipes since I was a graduate student in the early 1980s, which, according to my calculations, means I've lightened thousands of recipes!

Over the years, I've changed my focus to incorporate the latest nutrition science. For example, we now know that the type of fat we cook with is important, so I switch to "smart fats" whenever possible. I work to increase the fiber and nutrient content of recipes, just as I work to cut sodium and decrease calories from saturated fat and sugar.

Being "The Recipe Doctor" is part of my professional identity. I am honored to share my Recipe Doctor's 10 Heart Smart Cooking Commandments with you:

Recipe Doctor's 10 Heart Smart Cooking Commandments

1. In most bakery recipes (muffins, cakes, cookies, coffee cakes, bars, brownies, nut breads), you can substitute whole wheat flour for at least one-half of the white flour called for. Compared to 1/4 cup of white flour, each 1/4 cup of whole wheat flour adds 3.5 grams of fiber and various phytochemicals, and doubles the amount of magnesium and selenium. The extra fiber helps slow digestion and increase fullness.

2. In most bakery recipes, you can reduce the sugar called for by one-fourth without a big difference in taste and texture. So instead of adding 1 cup of sugar, you can add 3/4 cup. Or, if you like using Splenda, you can replace half of the sugar called for with Splenda (or a similar alternative sweetener approved for use in baking). This cuts 48 calories of sugar for every table-spoon you take out or replace with Splenda.

3. In egg dishes (quiches, frittatas, omelets, breakfast casseroles), you can use egg substitute or egg whites in place of half the eggs. In other words, if the recipe calls for six eggs, you would blend three whole eggs with 3/4 cup egg substitute (1/4 cup of egg substitute replaces each egg). You can replace half the eggs in bakery recipes with egg substitute as well. By replacing one large egg with 1/4 cup egg substitute, you'll shave 45 calories, 5 grams of fat, 1.6 grams of saturated fat, and 213 mg of cholesterol. If you don't like to use egg substitute products, you can also use egg whites for half of the eggs called for.

    When you are creating or lightening bakery recipes or batter, you can usually get away with only one egg because the emulsifying power of one egg yolk goes a long way. I usually add egg substitute or egg white to make up the difference so I'm still getting the protein from the eggs.

4. In many bakery recipes, you can cut the fat ingredient (butter, margarine, shortening, or oil) in half. So if a cake recipe calls for 1 cup of butter or margarine, you can usually use 1/2 cup instead. Remember to replace the missing fat with a similar amount of a moist but healthy ingredient (fat-free sour cream, orange juice, low-fat yogurt, applesauce, espresso). This change cuts both fat and calories, because each gram of fat translates into 9 calories as opposed to 4 calories for each gram of protein or carbohydrate.

   If you have found a light margarine with plant sterols that you like baking with, you can replace the total amount of fat called for in recipes directly with the light margarine. Most of these margarines already have about half of the fat per tablespoon, so adding them in the same amounts called for will cut the fat in half and boost your plant sterol intake.

5. Cook with reduced-fat or fat-free products when available—and when they taste good. Try fat-free sour cream, fat-free half-and-half, reduced-fat chees-es, light cream cheese, light mayonnaise, extra-lean meat without skin or visible fat, reduced-fat or light sausage, less-fat turkey bacon, light salad dressings, and light margarine for frosting. Many of these cut calories and saturated fat along with total fat. A few other fat-free products are in my arsenal as well: chicken broth, wine, strong coffee, fruit purees, and fruit juice. These foods add moisture, and sometimes flavor, to recipes instead of fatty ingredients.

6. Never deep-fry when you can oven-fry or pan-fry with a lot less oil. Choose canola oil or olive oil, and use about 1 teaspoon per serving (depending on the item). When you pan-fry or oven-fry in a controlled amount of oil, you can cut a lot of the fat and calories your food would soak up if it were submerged in hot oil. For every tablespoon of oil you cut, you'll save 120 calories and 13.5 grams of fat.

7. Use whole grains in your recipes whenever possible. We've already talked about whole wheat flour, but you can also substitute brown rice for white rice, add barley to stews and casseroles, and look for recipes that call for oats. There are also multigrain blends and whole wheat pastas to choose from in supermarkets. Whole grains offer a plethora of health benefits plus fiber to fill you up. One-fourth cup of dry brown rice contributes 2 grams of fiber, and a 2-ounce serving of dry multigrain spaghetti adds 4 grams or more of fiber to your diet.

8. Extra ingredients and embellishments can often be removed or cut in half. If a recipe calls for chocolate chips, you can use less. If it calls for dotting your casserole or pie with butter, you can skip this step. In a cake recipe, you can use half the original amount of frosting (in a double-layer cake, just frost the top and middle and forget the sides). With some cakes, bars, and cookies, you can skip the frosting in favor of a light sprinkling of powdered sugar. Using 2 tablespoons of frosting instead of 4 will shave off 130 calories, 4.5 grams of fat, and 2 grams of saturated fat. Each tablespoon of chocolate chips you skip cuts the calories by 50 per serving, the fat by 3 grams, and the saturated fat by almost 2 grams.

9. Use top-quality ingredients when possible. Start with the best-tasting, freshest ingredients you can find. Use fresh garlic and fresh herbs when you can. They usually have more flavor than the dried. Use ripe tomatoes and fresh lemons for zest or juice, extra-fresh fish, the sharpest reduced-fat Cheddar cheese, and so on.

10. Switch to "smart fat" ingredients when possible. Certain fats, when used in moderation, actually have health benefits. Omega-3 fatty acids (found in fish and some plant foods like canola oil and ground flaxseed), oils that contain monounsaturated fats (like olive and canola oil), and foods high in monounsaturated fats (like avocados and almonds) may help protect against heart disease. In recipes, you often have a choice of which oil or margarine to use. You can also add fish to some entree recipes instead of red meat.

Make the Switch to Canola and Olive Oil

When a recipe calls for *melted* butter or margarine, as in a chicken sautee, brownie, or pancake recipe, you can often substitute canola or olive oil.

Olive oil is highest in monounsaturated fat and contains some important phytochemicals (that come from olives), but it doesn't contribute any of the plant omega-3s. Canola oil is lowest in saturated fat of the cooking oils, contains an impressive amount of monounsaturated fat, and contributes the most plant omega-3s.

The U.S. Food and Drug Administration (FDA) recently approved a qualified health claim for canola oil that says, due to its unsaturated fat content, it may reduce the risk of coronary heart disease. (This is according to supportive, but not conclusive, research.) In 2004 the FDA approved a qualified health claim for olive oil regarding a reduced risk of coronary heart disease.

Caloric caution: At 9 calories per gram (1 gram of carbohydrate and protein contributes only 4 calories), you can have too much of a good thing even with smart fats—particularly if you are trying to lose some body weight. Switch to smart fats whenever possible, but keep things light: each tablespoon of oil contains around 120 calories.

The All-American Makeover

Even though America is a melting pot of people and cuisines, there are still foods and dishes that seem unmistakably American—ones that were created here or at least transformed into popular fare here. There are foods that may have been invented elsewhere but America made them into food phenomena all their own—french fries, fruit pies, cupcakes, popcorn, bagels, pizza, and the entire category of salads. There are foods that we put our own spin on, such as pancakes and waffles, grilled cheese sandwiches, and muffins. And, yes, there are foods that truly were invented on U.S. ground by Americans, such as Toll House chocolate chip cookies, corndogs, cornbread, doughnuts, potato chips, peanut butter and jelly sandwiches, and almost everything related to ice cream (ice cream sandwiches, hot fudge sundaes, root beer floats).

Don't get me wrong—these all-American foods are fantastic, and I celebrate wholeheartedly this culinary cornucopia that we live in. The problem is, most of these foods are energy dense, providing very few nutrients and grams of fiber, but a load of calories, saturated fat, total fat, sugar, and salt.

Some of these all-American foods are admittedly impossible to make over and still retain their desirable characteristics, like doughnuts. But so many others can be "doctored" to be lighter in calories, saturated fat, and sometimes sugar, and still stay true to the yummy quality that Americans have come to know and love.

The following are 10 tips for giving favorite American foods a heart smart makeover.

1. Apple Pie Makeover Tip: A lighter apple pie can be made with a lower fat, part whole wheat piecrust and by adding less sugar in the apple filling. No butter needs to "dot" the filling or the top crust either.

2. Chocolate Chip Cookie Makeover Tip: A lower-fat margarine with plant sterols can be used in place of a stick of butter or margarine. The sugar added can usually be decreased by one-fourth, and half of the white flour can be replaced with whole wheat flour. Using fewer chocolate chips will also shave off some calories and fat grams.

3. Cornbread Makeover Tip: Cornbread recipes can be lightened by using less fat in the batter. A less-fat margarine with plant sterols can be substituted for bacon grease, lard, or shortening. Replace the fat you remove with low-fat buttermilk or fat-free sour cream. In some recipes, a fat substitute blend can be made using canola oil and fat-free sour cream. Fewer eggs can be used: substitute 2 egg whites or 1/4 cup egg substitute for one of the eggs. If "stir-in" ingredients are called for, such as bacon or cheese, use reduced-fat options; you can also probably add less of them. Up the fiber in your cornbread by using whole wheat flour for half of the white flour.

4. Grilled Cheese Makeover Tip: A healthier grilled cheese sandwich can be made using whole wheat or multigrain bread (even multigrain sourdough bread) and reduced-fat cheese. Give the outer sides of the bread a quick spray of canola oil before placing on

your nonstick griddle or skillet, instead of slathering the bread with butter or margarine.

5. Muffin Makeover Tip: A nice muffin batter needs about 2 tablespoons of oil per 12 regular-sized muffins, and whole wheat flour can replace at least half of the white flour. Usually less sugar can be added, and ingredients like fresh or dried fruits, spices like ground cinnamon, and toasted nuts can boost the flavor.

6. Pancake Makeover Tip: Lighter pancakes can be made by using low-fat buttermilk or low-fat milk in the batter and adding very little fat (if any) to the skillet. But that's just half the health battle with pancakes. It's what people do to the pancakes after they are cooked that can calorically add up quickly. Keep the butter, whipped cream, and syrup to a minimum. If you like to use butter, use whipped butter (it's lower in fat per tablespoon and easier to spread and use less) and switch to reduced-calorie pancake syrup. Try topping your pancakes and waffles with fruit—it will add fiber and nutrients and will help give your stomach a satisfied feeling.

7. Pizza Makeover Tip: Look for the more authentic bread-like pizza crust recipes and replace half of the flour with whole wheat flour. Use lots of nutrient-rich pizza sauce, a moderate amount of reduced-fat cheese, and vegetables as toppings instead of high fat meat.

8. Fried Chicken Makeover Tip: Start with skinless chicken (half of the fat and saturated fat is in the skin) and add the seasoned flour coating or breadcrumb coating as preferred. Place the chicken pieces on a foil-lined baking sheet coated lightly with canola oil

(about 1/2 to 1 teaspoon per serving). Coat the top of the chicken with canola cooking spray. Bake in a 450-degree oven until the chicken is cooked through and coating is golden brown (about 25 minutes for breasts).

9. Potato Salad Makeover Tip: A light mayo dressing can be made using half light mayonnaise and half fat-free sour cream in place of regular mayonnaise. Punch up the flavor in the dressing with one or more of the following: honey mustard, relish, garlic, lemon juice, freshly ground black pepper, or other herbs and spices.

10. Fettuccine Alfredo Makeover Tip: Start by boiling whole wheat or whole grain blend pasta. To make a lower-fat white sauce, mix flour with twice as much fat-free half-and-half (for example 2 tablespoons flour blended with 1/4 cup of the half-and-half). Slowly whisk in the remaining fat-free half-and-half and then heat in saucepan until nicely thickened. Add black pepper or garlic as desired for flavor. Stir in some shredded Parmesan and combine with the pasta! We were able to completely eliminate the butter and the saturated fat coming from the cream or half-and-half.

40 Recipes to Get You Started

Since cooking at home is a key piece to heart-smart eating, I wanted to give you plenty of recipes to get you started in this direction. My recipes have all been tested, and were created with an eye on the nutrition content and an eye on the clock. These recipes are as nutritious and easy to prepare as practically possible.

All sorts of nutrition and diet suggestions have been thrown at you throughout this book. Here's where the buck stops. I put all of the guidelines and recommendations in a list, so they would be in one place. I kept these in mind as I developed the tasty recipes for this chapter.

Making sure you are getting enough:

- Omega-3s from fish: The American Heart Association suggests patients with documented coronary heart disease consume about 1 gram (or 1,000 mg) of EPA plus DHA per day, preferably from oily fish. Another way of looking at this is to eat fish, particularly oily fish, several times a week.

- Omega-3 (ALA) from plants: For ALA, a total intake of 1.5 to 3 grams per day seems beneficial, according to the American Heart Association. Include 1 to 2 tablespoons of ground flaxseed a day if it's okay with your cardiologist or doctor. Two tablespoons will contribute around 2.4 grams of omega-3s a day. Any other omega-3s you are getting from plants such as canola oil, walnuts, and soybeans would be in addition to this.

- Total and soluble fiber: I like to set the fiber "bar" at 25 grams per day (including about 10 or more grams of soluble fiber) because several studies noted that this is the amount that is particularly powerful.

- Polyphenol-rich plant foods: You can find nature's pharmaceuticals in plant foods such as whole grains, beans, nuts, fruits and vegetables, seeds, and red wine. Some of the standout plant foods that contribute two or more of the polyphenol phytochemicals are: purple grapes, tea, apples, berries, citrus fruits, nuts, and tomatoes.

Make sure you aren't getting too much:

- Saturated fat: Try not to get more than 7 percent of your calories from saturated fat. For someone eating around 2,000 calories a day, this would come out to no more than 16 grams a day; for someone eating about 2,500 calories, it would be less than 20 grams.

- Sodium: The latest research seems to suggest striving for no more than 1,500 mg of sodium a day.

- Total calories from fat: Even though a big part of eating heart smart is choosing the smart fats whenever possible and getting enough of the omega-3s, it is still important to eat an overall moderate fat diet. Some experts and agencies suggest getting no more than 25 percent of your calories from fat, with up to 9 percent of the total calories from polyunsaturated fat (which includes the omega-3s and omega-6 fatty acids).

- Calories: Anytime you can trim off empty calories from your diet or favorite recipes, it's a good thing— especially if you are trying to trim off extra weight around your midsection. The best way to keep calories away is to add less fat if a recipe calls for more than is really necessary. Each gram of fat contains 9 calories. Making cooking choices that lower saturated fat and sugar also tend to lower calories.

- Cholesterol from food: Try not to get more than 100 mg of cholesterol for every 1,000 calories you take in. For someone eating around 2,000 calories a day, this would be no more than 200 mg of cholesterol—the amount in one egg yolk. For someone eating 2,500 calories, the amount would increase to 250 mg a day.

Breakfast

High-Fiber Breakfast Bagel
Makes 1 serving

1 whole wheat bagel or English muffin

1 large egg, higher omega-3 (if available)

2 tablespoons egg substitute or 1 egg white

1 slice reduced-fat Cheddar cheese (about .75 ounce)

1. Place split bagel or English muffins in the toaster and toast until light brown.

2. Whisk egg and egg substitute or egg white together while heating a small nonstick saucepan over medium-high heat. Coat the bottom of the pan with canola cooking spray then pour in the egg mixture. Add a cover to the saucepan (this will cause the egg to puff up and cook on both sides).

3. Top the bottom bagel with the egg patty. Top the hot egg patty with a slice of reduced fat cheddar cheese. Place top half of the bagel over the cheese and enjoy!

Per serving: 294 calories, 22 g protein, 29 g carbohydrate, 10 g fat, 4.4 g saturated fat, 3 g monounsaturated fat, 2.5 g polyunsaturated fat, 240 mg cholesterol, 5 g fiber, 625 mg sodium. Calories from fat: 30 percent. Omega-3 fatty acids = .4 gram, Omega-6 fatty acids = .9 gram.

Breakfast Yogurt Parfait
Makes 1 serving

3/4 cup of lowfat vanilla or plain yogurt

1/2 cup fresh fruit (whatever is in season) such as blueberries, orange segments, etc.

1/2 cup whole grain breakfast cereal such as Grape Nuts, low-fat granola, or similar.

1 to 2 tablespoons chopped nuts (optional)

1. Combine yogurt with fresh fruit.

2. Top that with 1/2 cup whole grain breakfast cereal such as grape nuts, lowfat granola, or similar.

3. Sprinkle chopped nuts over the top if desired.

Per serving: 356 calories, 13 g protein, 65 g carbohydrate, 5.3 g fat, 2.1 g saturated fat, 2 g monounsaturated fat, 1 g polyunsaturated fat, 11 mg cholesterol, 5 g fiber, 255 mg sodium. Calories from fat: 13 percent. Omega-3 fatty acids = .2 gram, Omega-6 fatty acids = .8 gram.

Blueberry-Vanilla Walnut Almost-Instant Oatmeal
I know how convenient it is to have those instant oatmeal packets around. So here's a recipe that transforms a packet of instant oatmeal into blueberry bliss.

Makes 1 serving

1 packet plain instant oatmeal (or any compatible flavor such as Quaker Instant Oatmeal Nutrition for Women—Vanilla Cinnamon)*

2/3-cup lowfat milk (soy milk can also be used)

1/4 cup frozen blueberries (or 2 tablespoons dried blueberries)

1 tablespoon toasted walnut pieces

1. Empty packet into microwave-safe breakfast bowl. Stir in 2/3-cup milk and microwave on HIGH for 1 to 2 minutes.

2. Gently stir the blueberries into the oatmeal and top with a sprinkling of walnuts.

* If you don't use vanilla flavored instant oatmeal, stir 1/4-teaspoon vanilla extract into milk before you add it to the oats.

Per serving: 240 calories, 12 g protein, 32 g carbohydrate, 8 g fat, 1.7 g saturated fat, 2.1 g monounsaturated fat, 3.8 g polyunsaturated fat, 6 mg cholesterol, 4.3 g fiber, 370 mg sodium. Calories from fat: 29 percent. Omega-3 fatty acids = .7 gram, Omega-6 fatty acids = 3 grams.

Cranberry Pecan Oatmeal

This quick breakfast has one main ingredient that helps lower elevated serum cholesterol: oats. You can even stir in a couple teaspoons of ground flaxseed if you would like to make it a total of two lipid lowering ingredients! The pecans throw in some better fats, fiber, and some crunch, while the cranberries add some welcomed tang and color.

Makes 1 serving

1/2 cup Quick 1 Minute Oats

1 cup vanilla soy milk (1 cup lowfat milk + 1/4 teaspoon vanilla extract can be substituted)

2 tablespoons dried cranberries (i.e. Craisins) or other chopped dried fruit

1 tablespoon chopped roasted pecans, salted or unsalted

Dash salt (if using unsalted pecans)

2 teaspoons ground flaxseed (optional)

1 teaspoon white sugar (Splenda can be substituted)

1/4 teaspoon ground cinnamon

1. Combine the first six ingredients (oats, soy milk, cranberries, pecans, dash salt, and flaxseed if desired) in a medium, microwave-safe bowl.

2. Add the sugar and the cinnamon to a small custard cup and stir with fork to blend well; sprinkle over the oat mixture in the bowl.

3. Microwave on HIGH for 2 minutes; stir. Microwave on HIGH until most of the milk has been absorbed and oats appear to be softened (about 1 to 2 more minutes depending on your microwave and how well done you like your oatmeal).

Per serving: 280 calories, 12 g protein, 37 g carbohydrate, 9 g fat, 1.3 g saturated fat, 4.8 g monounsaturated fat, 2.9 g polyunsaturated fat, 0 mg cholesterol, 7 g fiber, 23 mg sodium. Calories from fat: 30 percent. Omega-3 fatty acids = .2 gram, Omega-6 fatty acids = 2.2 grams.

The "Cut Cholesterol" Fluffy Omelet

Eggs contain more than 200 mg of cholesterol per little yolk. There's nothing wrong with having an egg, but when you have a traditionally 2-egg entrée, I prefer to keep the cholesterol in the 200 mg ballpark (instead of 400) by using half eggs and half egg substitute. This just adds some protein from egg whites instead of the fats from the yolk. We also tend to add fatty ingredients to our egg dishes, so here's an omelet recipe where we cut everywhere we can but it still tastes delicious.

Makes 2 omelets

2 cups chopped broccoli florets

1/4 cup finely chopped pasilla pepper or green bell pepper

4 green onions, sliced diagonally

1 1/2 teaspoons minced or chopped garlic

1 cup low sodium chicken broth

2 large eggs, separated (higher omega-3 eggs if available)

1/2 cup egg substitute

Canola cooking spray

Pepper to taste

Herbs and salt-free herb blends if desired

1/4 cup reduced-fat shredded sharp cheddar cheese

1. Coat a medium nonstick frying pan with canola oil cooking spray. Add broccoli, pepper, green onions, and garlic and cook over medium heat about 1 minute, stirring frequently. Pour in chicken broth and cook, stirring frequently, until vegetables are tender (broth probably will have evaporated).

2. Add egg yolks and egg substitute to a small mixing bowl and beat on low speed until smooth; set aside. Whip egg whites with electric mixer until stiff. Fold the egg whites carefully into egg yolk mixture.

3. Generously coat a nonstick omelet or medium frying pan with canola cooking spray (or use 1/2 teaspoon canola oil) while starting to heat the pan over medium heat.

4. Spread half of the egg mixture into the pan so the egg mixture fills the bottom of the pan. Sprinkle the top with pepper to taste or any herbs or salt-free herb blends you desire. Cover pan to help cook the top.

5. After a minute or two, the bottom should be nicely browned and the top should be firm. Add half of the vegetable mixture to half of the omelet (to make a half circle). Sprinkle half of the cheese over the vegetables. Flip the unfilled half over and remove to a serving plate.

6. Repeat with remaining egg mixture, vegetable mixture, and cheese.

Per serving: 193 calories, 21 g protein, 10 g carbohydrate, 8 g fat, 3.7 g saturated fat, 2.6 g monounsaturated fat, 1.5 g polyunsaturated fat, 223 mg cholesterol, 4 g fiber, 318 mg sodium. Calories from fat: 37 percent. Omega-3 fatty acids = .5 gram, Omega-6 fatty acids = 1 gram.

Applesauce Spice Muffins

The oat bran, applesauce, and flaxseed in these muffins give the soluble fiber a big boost. The flaxseed and canola oil also add some plant omega-3s into the picture.

Makes 12 muffins

1/2 cup oat bran

1/4 cup ground flaxseed

1/2 cup unbleached white flour

1/2 cup whole wheat flour

1 1/2 teaspoons baking powder

1/2 teaspoon baking soda

1/2 teaspoon ground cinnamon

1/2 teaspoon ground allspice

1/4 teaspoon ground nutmeg

1/4 teaspoon salt

1 large egg, higher omega-3 if available

1/4 cup egg substitute

2/3 cup brown sugar, packed

3 tablespoons canola oil

1/2 cup lowfat buttermilk

1 cup unsweetened applesauce

1/2 cup coarsely chopped pecans or walnuts (optional)

1. Preheat oven to 400 degrees. Line muffin cups with foil or paper liners.

2. Add oat bran, flaxseed, flour, baking powder, baking soda, cinnamon, allspice, nutmeg, and salt to a large bowl and whisk together until well blended.

3. Add egg, egg substitute, and brown sugar to a large mixing bowl and beat on medium speed until combined. Add the canola oil and buttermilk and beat on medium speed until the mixture is creamy. Beat in the applesauce on low speed until combined.

4. Gradually beat in the flour mixture, while mixer is on low speed, just until combined. Stir in the nuts if desired. Fill prepared muffin cups with about 1/4 cup of batter each.

5. Bake until tester inserted in center comes out clean (about 20 to 25 minutes).

Per muffin: 142 calories, 4 g protein, 22 g carbohydrate, 5 g fat, .5 g saturated fat, 2.5 g monounsaturated fat, 1.8 g polyunsaturated fat, 18 mg cholesterol, 3 g fiber, 186 mg sodium. Calories from fat: 31 percent. Omega-3 fatty acids = 1 gram, Omega-6 fatty acids = .8 gram.

Spinach Quiche Muffins
Spinach is rich in the three minerals that help lower blood pressure and is also one of the higher omega-3 plant foods.

Makes 12 muffins

1 3/4 cups lowfat milk or fat-free half and half, divided use

2 large eggs (higher omega-3 eggs if available)

1/2 cup egg substitute

1/8 teaspoon white pepper

1/8 teaspoon ground nutmeg

1/2 cup whole wheat flour (unbleached white can be substituted)

10-ounce box frozen spinach, thawed, gently squeezed of extra moisture, and coarsely chopped with a knife (about 1 cup)

1 1/2 cups reduced-fat shredded sharp cheddar or Swiss cheese, packed

1/3 cup finely shredded Parmesan cheese

1. Preheat oven to 350 degrees. Coat muffin pan generously with canola cooking spray.

2. Beat 1 1/4 cup of the milk with the eggs; egg substitute, pepper, and nutmeg.

3. Combine remaining 1/2 cup of milk with flour to make a paste. Beat paste into egg mixture until smooth.

4. Stir in spinach and both cheeses.

5. Fill each muffin cup with 1/4 cup of batter. Bake until cooked throughout (about 12 to 15 minutes).

Per serving: 112 calories, 10 g protein, 8 g carbohydrate, 5 g fat, 2.9 g saturated fat, 1 g monounsaturated fat, 1 g polyunsaturated fat, 40 mg cholesterol, 2 g fiber, 225 mg sodium. Calories from fat: 40 percent. Omega-3 fatty acids = .2 gram, Omega-6 fatty acids = .8 gram.

Blueberry Blast Smoothie/Shake

This is a fun, refreshing way to work a serving of lowfat milk and yogurt and phytochemical-rich blueberries into your day. I keep a bag of frozen blueberries in the freezer just so I can make this smoothie!

Makes 1 serving

1/3 cup light or lowfat vanilla ice-cream or lowfat frozen yogurt

2/3 cup frozen blueberries

1/4 cup blueberry lowfat yogurt (other berry flavored yogurt can be used)

1/4 cup lowfat milk

1/2 teaspoon vanilla extract

1 tablespoon ground flaxseed (optional)

1. Add all ingredients to a blender and blend on medium speed until mixture is smooth.

2. Add to serving cup and enjoy with a spoon or straw!

Per serving: 201 calories, 8 g protein, 37 g carbohydrate, 3 g fat, 1.5 g saturated fat, 1 g monounsaturated fat, .5 g polyunsaturated fat, 20 mg cholesterol, 3 g fiber, 130 mg sodium. Calories from fat: 20 percent. Omega-3 fatty acids = .1 gram, Omega-6 fatty acids = .4 gram.

Side Dishes

All American Light (No Boil) Potato Salad
Makes about 6 cups of salad (8, 3/4-cup servings)

4 russet potatoes with skin (large pink or white potatoes can be substituted)

1/4 cup light mayonnaise

1/4 cup fat-free sour cream

1 tablespoon honey mustard (add 1 more tablespoon if desired)

1/4 teaspoon black pepper

1/2 teaspoon salt (optional)

1/2 cup diced or chopped celery

1/3 cup diced or chopped red bell pepper

1/3 cup chopped green onions

1 tablespoon fresh chopped parsley (regular or Italian)

1/2 teaspoon paprika (optional)

1. Wash the outside of potatoes well then cut into 1-inch cubes. Add potato pieces to a large microwave-safe container. Cover and cook on HIGH for about 6 minutes. Stir potatoes, cover container, and cook on HIGH until potatoes are just tender (about 4-6 minutes more).

2. While potatoes are cooling, add mayonnaise, sour cream, honey mustard, pepper, and salt (if desired) to large bowl and whisk to combine.

3. Stir in cooled potatoes, celery, bell pepper, green onions, and parsley. Cover and chill until ready to serve (at least an hour). Sprinkle a dash or two of paprika over the top before serving if desired.

Per serving: 148 calories, 3 g protein, 29 g carbohydrate, 2.4 g fat, .3 g saturated fat, 1.3 g monounsaturated fat, .8 g polyunsaturated fat, 0 mg cholesterol, 3 g fiber, 89 mg sodium (216 mg if the salt is added). Calories from fat: 14 percent. Omega-3 fatty acids = .1 g, Omega-6 fatty acids = .7 gram.

Cilantro Brown Rice
Makes 4 to 6 servings

1 cup uncooked brown rice

2 cups water

1/2 cup fresh cilantro leaves

1/2 cup fresh spinach leaves

1/4 cup fresh chopped scallions (or green onions)

2 tablespoon fresh parsley leaves

4 teaspoons canola oil

1/4 teaspoon salt

1/4 teaspoon pepper

1. Add brown rice and water to rice cooker (or cook rice over the stove following directions on bag of rice).

2. While rice cooks, in small food processor bowl, pulse together cilantro, spinach, scallions, parsley, canola oil, salt, and pepper until finely chopped.

3. When rice has finished cooking, transfer hot cooked rice from the rice cooker into medium serving bowl and fluff rice with a fork. Add cilantro pesto to cooked rice and stir gently until combined well. Cover bowl and let rest for about 5 minutes. Serve!

Per serving (if 6 per recipe): 145 calories, 3 g protein, 24 g carbohydrate, 4 g fat, .4 g saturated fat, 2 g monounsaturated fat, 1.2 g polyunsaturated fat, 0 mg cholesterol, 1.5 g fiber, 103 mg sodium. Calories from fat: 25 percent. Omega-3 fatty acids = .3 gram, Omega-6 fatty acids = .9 gram.

Light Waldorf Salad
Makes about 6 1/2 cups (6 servings)

3/4 cup plain lowfat yogurt

2 teaspoons honey

1 teaspoon lemon zest, finely chopped

2 large apples, peeled, cored, and chopped (about 3 cups)

2 cups red seedless grapes

1 cup thinly sliced celery

1/3 cup toasted walnut pieces

1/3 cup dried fruit like raisins, cherries or cranberries (optional)

1. In serving bowl, combine yogurt, honey and lemon zest together with whisk.

2. Add apple pieces, grapes, celery, walnuts, and dried fruit if desired and toss everything together. Cover and chill in refrigerator until ready to serve.

Per serving: 138 calories, 4 g protein, 22 g carbohydrate, 4.6 g fat, .6 g saturated fat, 1.3 g monounsaturated fat, 2.5 g polyunsaturated fat, 3 mg cholesterol, 3 g fiber, 36 mg sodium. Calories from fat: 30 percent. Omega-3 fatty acids = .2 gram, Omega-6 fatty acids = 2.3 grams.

Quick Fix Tabbouleh Salad
This is one of most popular ways to use bulgur.

Makes 6 servings

1 cup dry bulgur

1 cup boiling water

3/4 teaspoon low sodium chicken broth powder (vegetable broth powder can be substituted)

1/4 cup toasted walnut pieces (pecans can be substituted)

1/2 cup chopped green onions, white and part green

1 1/2 cups diced fresh tomatoes (or 10 cherry tomatoes, quartered)

3 tablespoons lemon juice

2 tablespoons olive oil

Pepper to taste

1. Pour boiling water over bulgur in 8 cup measure (or medium-sized bowl) and let sit 30 minutes (until water is absorbed).

2. Blend 3/4 teaspoon chicken broth powder with 3 table-spoons very hot water together in custard cup and set aside.

3. Add remaining ingredients including chicken broth, pine nuts, green onions, tomatoes, lemon juice, and olive oil. Toss thoroughly and add pepper to taste. Cover and chill at least 2 hours.

Per serving: 169 calories, 5.5 g protein, 21 g carbohydrate, 7.2 g fat, .8 g saturated fat, 4 g monounsaturated fat, 2.5 g polyunsaturated fat, 0 mg cholesterol, 5.5 g fiber, 17 mg sodium. Calories from fat: 38 percent. Omega-3 fatty acids = .2 gram, Omega-6 fatty acids = 2.3 grams.

Sunshine Salad

You'll get plenty of vitamin A and C from the spinach, oranges, and strawberries when you have a serving of this salad!

Makes 2 to 4 servings

4 cups fresh spinach

1 cup orange segments or sliced nectarines or peaches (peeled)

1 cup fresh sliced or halved strawberries

4 tablespoons light or reduced-calorie Italian dressing or light raspberry vinaigrette (made with olive or canola oil)

2 tablespoons roasted sunflower seeds

1. Toss spinach, fruit, and dressing together.

2. Sprinkle sunflower seeds on top.

3. Spoon into four salad bowls and enjoy!

Per serving (if 4 per recipe): 87 calories, 2.3 g protein, 13 g carbohydrate, 3 g fat (.2 g saturated fat, 1 g monounsaturated fat, 1.6 g polyunsaturated fat), 0 mg cholesterol, 3 g fiber, 184 mg sodium. Calories from fat: 30 percent. Omega-3 fatty acids = .2 gram, Omega-6 fatty acids = 1.4 gram.

Salad Nicoise

This dish contains two items that help lower blood pressure—omega-3 fatty acids from the tuna and kidney beans, and vegetables.

Makes 6 servings

3 medium potatoes

3 large hard boiled eggs (the yolks will be thrown away later)

2 medium tomatoes

13 ounce can of albacore tuna, canned in water, drained

3/4 cup artichoke hearts, bottled in water, rinsed, well drained, and chopped

1 cup lower sodium kidney beans, drained and rinsed

About 18 Spanish or black olives, pitted (about 1/2 cup)

8 cups shredded Romaine lettuce

Dressing:

3 tablespoons olive oil

1/4 cup red wine vinegar

1/3 cup apple juice

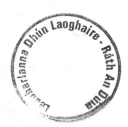

2 tablespoons honey

1/8 teaspoon black pepper

1/2 teaspoon dried chervil

1/2 teaspoon dried tarragon

1. Cook potatoes in microwave until fork-tender. Refrigerate potatoes and hard-boiled eggs until chilled.

2. Cut potatoes into bite-size pieces and place in medium-sized serving bowl. Peel eggs under running cold water; cut each egg into 4 wedges. Discard the egg yolks. Place egg whites in a large serving bowl.

3. Cut tomatoes into wedges and add to serving bowl. Separate tuna into bite-size pieces and add to serving bowl along with artichoke hearts, beans, and olives.

4. Add dressing ingredients to a small food processor or blender; process until well blended and smooth. Pour into serving bowl and toss well with tuna, egg white wedges, and vegetables.

5. Place about 2 cups of lettuce on each plate. Spoon a good portion of the mixture over lettuce.

Per serving: 319 calories, 22 g protein, 38 g carbohydrate, 9 g fat, 1.5 g saturated fat, 6.1 g monounsaturated fat, 1.4 g polyunsaturated fat, 22 mg cholesterol, 7.3 g fiber, 345 mg sodium. Calories from fat: 27 percent. Omega-3 fatty acids = .3 gram, Omega-6 fatty acids = 1 gram.

Brussels Sprouts With Pecans and Shallots

I love that this dish is pretty easy to throw together but looks interesting and elegant on a holiday table.

Makes 8 servings

8 cups brussels sprout halves (trim off end of each sprout and cut in half)

4 strips turkey bacon

1 tablespoon canola oil

1 cup sliced shallots

1 teaspoon minced garlic

3/4 cup pecan pieces, lightly toasted in a nonstick frying pan

2 teaspoons brown sugar

1. Micro-steam the brussels sprouts with a couple tablespoons of water until just barely tender (about 6 minutes, depending on your microwave). Watch carefully so they don't overcook. Drain them from any excess water.

2. Meanwhile, cook the turkey bacon strips over medium-high heat in a large nonstick frying pan coated with canola cooking spray, flipping them often, until crisp. Let them cool on a paper towel and then break them into small pieces.

3. Add the canola oil to the same pan from the turkey bacon and heat over a medium-high flame. Add the shallots and sauté, stirring frequently, for a couple of minutes.

4. Add the minced garlic and sauté another minute or two or until the shallots are golden.

5. Stir in the brussels sprout halves and sauté a couple of minutes, stirring occasionally, to char part of the sprouts.

6. Sprinkle pecans and brown sugar over the top and stir to blend. Reduce heat to medium-low and continue to cook and stir for another minute. Add salt and pepper to taste if desired.

7. Spoon the mixture into a serving bowl and sprinkle turkey bacon bits over the top.

Per serving: 165 calories, 6 g protein, 20 g carbohydrate, 9 g fat, .9 g saturated fat, 5.2 g monounsaturated fat, 3 g polyunsaturated fat, 6 mg cholesterol, 5 g fiber, 110 mg sodium. Calories from fat: 49 percent. Omega-3 fatty acids = .4 gram, Omega-6 fatty acids = 2.6 grams.

Homemade Lentil Soup

If you are trying to eat more beans, lentil soup is a good place to start. Because of this tiny size, they can cook up from a dry bean in about 30 minutes.

Makes 8 large soup servings

2 cups chopped onions

4 teaspoons minced or crushed garlic

3 tablespoons olive oil

8 cups low-sodium chicken broth

1 pound dried lentils, washed and picked over

2 potatoes, washed and diced

4 Roma tomatoes, quartered

2 large carrots, diced

2 tablespoons fresh oregano leaves, finely chopped (or 1 1/2 teaspoon dried oregano leaves)

3/4 teaspoon freshly ground black pepper

Salt and pepper to taste (optional)

1. In a large saucepan, sauté the onion and garlic in olive oil until lightly browned. Add all other ingredients and bring to a boil. Cover and let soup boil for 15 minutes.

2. Lower heat to a simmer and let cook around 30 to 60 minutes.

Per serving: 354 calories, 22 g protein, 53 g carbohydrate, 8 g fat, 1.8 g saturated fat, 3.9 g monounsaturated fats, .8 g polyunsaturated fat, 5 mg cholesterol, 11 g fiber, 133 mg sodium. Calories from fat: 19 percent. Omega-3 fatty acids = 1 gram, Omega-6 fatty acids = .7 gram.

Tuscan Vegetable Soup

This is a wonderful vegetable soup full of an assortment of winter-time veggies.

Makes 12 small bowls of soup (or 6 very large bowls)

1 tablespoon olive oil

1 1/2 cups finely chopped onion (about 1 large)

1 1/2 teaspoons dried thyme (2 tablespoons of chopped fresh thyme can be used)

3 teaspoons minced garlic

4 cups coarsely chopped green cabbage

14.5-ounce can Italian style stewed tomatoes

2 cups sliced celery

2 cups diced (1/2-inch pieces) carrots or baby carrots

8 cups low sodium chicken broth (vegetable broth can be substituted)

3 cups diced (1/2-inch pieces) potato

1/2 cup chopped fresh basil

3 cups half-slices of zucchini (cut zucchini in half then cut into slices)

15 ounce can red kidney beans (white kidney beans—cannellini can be substituted), rinsed and drained

Optional garnish: Shredded Parmesan cheese (about a tablespoon per serving)

1. Heat olive oil in large, nonstick saucepan over medium heat. Add in the onion, thyme, and garlic and sauté about 3 to 5 minutes.

2. Stir in the cabbage pieces, the can of stewed tomatoes (including liquid), celery, and carrots and sauté 8-10 minutes. Stir in the chicken broth, potatoes, fresh basil, zucchini, and kidney beans and bring back to a boil. Reduce heat to simmer, cover saucepan, and let simmer about 1 hour.

3. Spoon into soup bowls and top each serving with a tablespoon of Parmesan cheese.

Per small bowl serving: 138 calories, 7 g protein, 24 g carbohydrate, 3 g fat, .9 g saturated fat, 1.5 g monounsaturated fat, .6 g polyunsaturated fat, 3 mg cholesterol, 7 g fiber, 113 mg sodium. Calories from fat: 17 percent. Omega-3 fatty acids = .15 gram, Omega-6 fatty acid = .45 gram.

Honey & Oat Bread (for bread machine)
This is a great bread for making toast or sandwiches.

Makes 12 slices

1 cup rolled oats

1 cup lowfat buttermilk

1 large egg (higher omega-3 if available), beaten

2 tablespoons hot tap water

2 tablespoons honey

2 tablespoons canola oil

1 cup whole wheat flour

1 1/2 cups unbleached white flour

1 teaspoon salt

2 teaspoons active dry yeast

1. Add oats to food processor and pulse to create a flour like mixture.

2. Add buttermilk, beaten egg, hot water, honey, canola oil, flours, salt, and yeast to the bread machine pan in this order or the order suggested by the manufacturer.

3. Set the bread machine on the Light Crust or Whole Wheat setting and press START. The bread will be ready in about 4 hours.

Per serving: 168 calories, 6 g protein, 28 g carbohydrate, 3.8 g fat, .5 g saturated fat, 1.8 g monounsaturated fat, 1 g polyunsaturated fat, 18 mg cholesterol, 2.1 g fiber, 230 mg sodium. Calories from fat: 20 percent. Omega-3 fatty acids = .2 gram, Omega-6 fatty acid = .8 gram.

Lunches and Light Dinner Entrees

Chicken Pesto Pine Nut Skillet Pizza
Makes 1 large serving or 2 small servings

2 multi-grain flour tortillas

1 tablespoon pesto sauce

1/2 cup shredded roasted or grilled chicken breast, skinless

2 slices part-skim mozzarella (2 ounces), each broken into about 4 pieces

1 tablespoon toasted pine nuts (pignolis)

1. Add a flour tortilla to a large, nonstick frying pan over medium-high heat. Spread pesto on top of the tortilla then top with chicken and then cheese and pine nuts.

2. Place the second tortilla on top and once the bottom tortilla is nicely browned, carefully flip the pizza over to brown the other tortilla. This will take about a minute or two more.

3. Remove pizza to a plate and cut pizza into 8 wedges.

Per large serving: 570 calories, 45 g protein, 48 g carbohydrate, 21 g fat, 9 g saturated fat, 5 g monounsaturated fat, 6 g polyunsaturated fat, 78 mg cholesterol, 11 g fiber, 1300 mg sodium. Calories from fat: 33 percent. Omega-3 fatty acids = .3 gram, Omega-6 fatty acids = 5 grams.

Topless Chicken Pot Pie

Break your addiction to frozen pot pies with this recipe for topless chicken pot pie. If you want to trim some prep time, substitute 1 2/3 cups Bertolli Mushroom Alfredo (bottled) for the homemade white sauce. You can also make this dish with or without the bottom crust.

Makes 5 servings

1 whole wheat piecrust, uncooked (crust is optional)

Filling:

2 teaspoons olive oil or canola oil

3/4 cup chopped onion

3/4 cup chopped or sliced celery

3/4 cup chopped carrot (baby carrots can be used)

1 teaspoon minced or chopped garlic

3 cups roasted or grilled skinless and boneless chicken breast, diced

Homemade White Sauce Option:

1/2 cup light cream cheese

1 cup fat-free half and half

1 tablespoon unbleached white flour

1/4 teaspoon ground white or black pepper

Topping:

1/3 cup panko crumbs

1/3 cup quick or old-fashioned oats

1/3 cup shredded Parmesan cheese

2 teaspoons parsley flakes

Olive oil or canola cooking spray

1. Preheat oven to 400 degrees. Set piecrust, if desired, in a 9-inch, deep-dish pie pan (if not already in one) or divide crust into five equal circles if using individual pot pie dishes. If making individual pot pies, place each of the crust circles into an individual dish or ramekin about 4- to 4.5-inches wide, set aide.

2. Pour 2 teaspoons oil into a medium nonstick saucepan over medium-high heat. When hot, stir in the onion, celery, and carrot and sauté for a few minutes. Stir in the garlic and continue to sauté for another minute. Scoop this mixture into a medium bowl and set aside.

3. Combine light cream cheese, half and half, and flour in a small food processor (or electric mixer) pulsing until smooth.

4. In same medium saucepan over medium-high heat, pour in the cream cheese mixture and continue to stir and gently boil until it thickens (about 2 minutes).

5. Turn off the heat and stir in the pepper, sautéed vegetables, and diced chicken. Spoon mixture into the crust lined pie plate or if making individual pot pies, divide the filling between the five individual dishes (about 1 1/4 cups).

6. For the topping, in medium sized bowl, combine the Panko, oats, and Parmesan cheese and parsley flakes. Spread topping over the top of the large pot pie or five small pot pies.

7. Coat the top generously with canola or olive oil cooking spray. Place pot pie(s) on a cookie sheet and bake in oven for about 30 minutes (for one large pie) or 20 minutes (for individual pies), or until crust is nicely browned.

Per serving (with bottom crust): 440 calories, 36 g protein, 33 g carbohydrate, 18 g fat, 7 g saturated fat, 7 g monounsaturated fat, 2 g polyunsaturated fat, 93 mg cholesterol, 5 g fiber, 564 mg sodium. Calories from fat: 36 percent. Omega-3 fatty acids = .2 gram, Omega-6 fatty acids = 1.6 gram.

Per serving (without bottom crust): 320 calories, 35 g protein, 18 g carbohydrate, 11 g fat, 5 g saturated fat, 3 g monounsaturated fat, 1 g polyunsaturated fat, 93 mg cholesterol, 2 g fiber, 401 mg sodium. Calories from fat: 31 percent. Omega-3 fatty acids = .1 gram, Omega-6 fatty acids = .6 gram.

Chicken Enchilada Casserole

I was able to cut the total fat and saturated fat in half and lower the calories by 150 per serving by doing a few simple things.

Makes 8 servings

4 cups shredded, roasted, skinless chicken breast (about 4 chicken breast halves)

1 cup chopped onion

12 corn tortillas (each torn into 4 pieces—to absorb the sauce better)

32 ounces green chili enchilada sauce or bottled salsa Verde (red enchilada sauce can be substituted if desired)

8 ounce package reduced-fat shredded Monterey Jack cheese (or mixture of reduced fat Jack and cheddar cheeses), about 2 cups

8 ounces fat-free sour cream (light sour cream may also be used)

1. Preheat oven to 350 degrees. Coat a 9 x 13-inch baking dish with canola cooking spray.

2. Pour about 1 cup of enchilada sauce in the bottom of the prepared baking dish. Arrange four tortillas in a single layer in pan. Top with 1/2 of the shredded chicken, 1/2 of the onion, 1/3 of the shredded cheese, and 1/2 cup of the sour cream. Use a spatula to spread the sour cream in the pan, and then top with a cup of the enchilada sauce.

3. Repeat the layers starting with four tortillas broken up into four pieces each, then the remaining chicken, onion, another third of the cheese, and remaining sour cream. Use a spatula to spread the sour cream in the pan, and then top with a cup of enchilada sauce.

4. Top with remaining four tortillas, remaining enchilada sauce (about 3/4 cup) and remaining shredded cheese.

5. Coat one side of a sheet of foil with canola cooking spray and cover the pan with the foil (coated side down—this keeps the cheese from sticking to the foil) and bake for 45 minutes.

Per serving: 307 calories, 27 g protein, 33 g carbohydrate, 7.5 g fat (4 g saturated fat, 2 g monounsaturated fat, 1.5 g polyunsaturated fat), 54 mg cholesterol, 4 g fiber, 598 mg sodium. Calories from fat: 22 percent. Omega-3 fatty acids = .1 gram, Omega-6 fatty acids = 1.4 grams.

Chicken Parmesan Pizza
Makes 4 servings

1 1/2 cups bottled pizza sauce (marinara sauce can be substituted)

2 cups shredded, skinless, roasted chicken breast

1 1/2 cups shredded part-skim mozzarella

1/2 cup shredded Parmesan cheese

1/3 cup chopped green onions (white and part of green)

Bread Machine Pizza Crust:

3/4 cup + 1 teaspoon warm water

1 1/2 tablespoons olive oil

2 teaspoons minced garlic

1/2 cup oat bran

1/2 cup whole wheat flour

1 cup unbleached white flour

1/2 cup salt

1 teaspoon sugar

1 packet rapid rise or active dry yeast (1/2 ounce or 2 teaspoons)

1. Place ingredients in bread machine pan in the order recommended by the manufacturer. Close the lid and select the DOUGH cycle (usually 1 hour 40 minutes), and press START.

2. At the end of the cycle, remove dough from pan, dust the dough lightly with flour, and let rest 15 minutes. Meanwhile preheat oven to 400 degrees. Stretch dough out to fit your pizza pan (about 14-inch round or 9 x 13-inch rectangle).

3. Spread 1 1/2 cups of pizza sauce over the top of the dough and arrange chicken on top of the sauce. Sprinkle mozzarella and Parmesan cheese and green onions (if desired) over the top. Bake for 15 to 20 minutes or until the crust is lightly browned on the bottom and the cheese is nice and bubbly.

Per serving: 550 calories, 45 g protein, 54 g carbohydrate, 16 g fat, 7 g saturated fat, 7 g monounsaturated fat, 2 g polyunsaturated fat, 88 mg cholesterol, 7 g fiber, 900 mg sodium. Calories from fat: 26 percent. Omega-3 fatty acids = 0 gram, Omega-6 fatty acids = 2 grams.

Apple-Walnut Albacore Tuna Salad

Canned albacore tuna is a terrific and convenient source of omega-3 fatty acids found in fish. This is a light, sweet and crunchy rendition of the standby tuna salad sandwich.

Makes 2 sandwiches

6 1/4 ounce can Albacore tuna canned in water, drained well

1 small apple, cored and finely chopped

2 tablespoons toasted walnut pieces (baked or broiled until lightly brown)

1 tablespoon light mayonnaise

1 tablespoon fat free sour cream

1/8 teaspoon ground cinnamon

1 tablespoon apple juice or cider

4 slices of whole wheat or whole grain bread

Lettuce leaves

1. Add tuna, apple, and walnut pieces to medium serving bowl and toss.

2. Blend mayonnaise with sour cream, cinnamon, and apple juice. Combine this dressing with the tuna mixture.

3. Spread half of the tuna mixture onto a slice of bread and top with lettuce leaves and a second slice of bread. Repeat with remaining tuna, lettuce, and bread to make a second sandwich.

Per serving: 390 calories, 29.5 g protein, 47 g carbohydrate, 10 g fat, 1.7 g saturated fat, 2.3 g monounsaturated fat, 4 g polyunsaturated fat, 23 mg cholesterol, 7 g fiber, 693 mg sodium. Calories from fat: 24 percent. Omega-3 fatty acids = .6 gram, Omega-6 fatty acids = 3.4 grams.

Seafood and Spinach Fettuccine with Lemon Rosemary Sauce
Makes 4 servings

8 ounces dried whole wheat or whole-wheat blend fettuccine or spaghetti noodles

2 tablespoons unbleached white flour or Wondra flour

1 cup fat-free half and half

4 cups fresh spinach, packed

1 cup double strength chicken broth, divided into 1/4 cup and 3/4 cup

1 tablespoon whipped butter, reduced-fat margarine, or canola oil

1/3 cup chopped shallots

2 tablespoons lemon juice (juice from 1 large lemon)

Zest from 1 large lemon, finely chopped

3/4 cup double strength chicken broth

2 teaspoons chopped fresh rosemary

Freshly ground black pepper to taste

6 ounces grilled or cooked salmon cut into small pieces or 4 ounces lox cut into small pieces (or 12 ounces cooked shrimp—peeled and deveined)

1/4 cup shredded Parmesan cheese (optional)

1. Start boiling pasta as directed on the package. When ready, drain noodles and set aside.

2. In a small bowl, combine 2 tablespoons of flour with 1/4 cup of the fat-free half and half. Stir in the remaining fat-free half and half and set aside.

3. In medium nonstick saucepan, cook spinach down over medium heat with 1/4-cup chicken broth (about 2 minutes). Spoon into bowl and set aside.

4. Add a tablespoon of margarine, whipped butter, or canola oil to the medium nonstick saucepan and sauté the shallots for about 2 minutes over medium heat. Stir in 2 tablespoons of lemon juice and the zest from 1 lemon, 3/4-cup double strength chicken broth, fresh rosemary, and the fat-free half and half mixture.

5. Continue to simmer this mixture until nicely thickened. Turn heat off and add black pepper to taste.

6. Stir in the spinach and seafood of choice (salmon, lox, or shrimp). Cover and let dish rest for a couple of minutes to blend flavors.

7. Spoon each serving of the seafood and spinach mixture over drained, cooked fettuccine or spaghetti noodles. Sprinkle a tablespoon of Parmesan cheese over each serving if desired.

Per serving (with grilled salmon): 369 calories, 23 g protein, 55 g carbohydrate, 7 g fat, 2.4 g saturated fat, 2.1 g monounsaturated fat, 2 g polyunsaturated fat, 40 mg cholesterol, 7 g fat, 434 mg sodium. Calories from fat: 17 percent. Omega-3 fatty acids = 1.2 grams, Omega-6 fatty acids = .6 grams.

Seafood Salad
Makes 3 servings

2 tablespoons light mayonnaise

1/3 cup fat-free or light sour cream

Juice from 1/2 lemon

1 cup shredded, cooked crabmeat or imitation crabmeat (about 1/3 pound)

1 cup bay shrimp (cooked), about 1/3 pound

1/2 cup chopped celery

1/4 teaspoon salt (optional)

1/4 teaspoon freshly ground pepper (add more to taste)

2 tablespoons sliced black olives

1 green onion, chopped

6 cups chopped Romaine, spinach, or green leaf lettuce

1. Combine light mayonnaise with sour cream and lemon juice in medium sized bowl.

2. Stir in crab, shrimp, celery, salt if desired, pepper, olives, and green onions. Chill at least 1 hour.

3. Serve each serving of seafood salad on a bed of 2 cups of lettuce greens.

Per serving: 180 calories, 22 g protein, 9.3 g carbohydrate, 5.8 g fat, .9 g saturated fat, 1.7 g monounsaturated fat, 2.7 g polyunsaturated fat, 139 mg cholesterol, 2 g fiber, 343 mg sodium. Calories from fat: 29 percent. Omega-3 fatty acids = .5 gram, Omega-6 fatty acids = 2 grams.

Light Salmon Fritters
Makes 3 servings (about 3 fritters each)

1 egg yolk (from omega-3 egg if available)

2 tablespoons egg substitute

2 tablespoons flour

1/4 teaspoon salt

1/4 teaspoon dill weed

1/8 teaspoon pepper

1/2 teaspoon parsley flakes (or 1 teaspoon chopped fresh parsley)

1 3/4 to 2 cups de-boned, de-skinned, and poached or grilled salmon—preferably wild—broken into very small pieces

2 egg whites

Canola cooking spray

1. Beat egg yolk with egg substitute in medium sized bowl until thick. Add flour, salt, dill, pepper, and parsley, and stir to blend. Stir salmon pieces into flour mixture.

2. Beat egg whites until stiff. Fold them into salmon mixture.

3. Coat a nonstick frying pan generously with canola cooking spray. Start heating the pan over medium heat.

4. Scoop out 1/4 cup of the fritter batter and add to pan. Repeat with remaining batter until pan is full. Continue to cook until bottom side is nicely browned (about 3 to 5 minutes). Turn to other side and cook until browned (3 minutes more)

5. Remove fritters from pan and repeat step 4 to finish the fritter batter.

Per serving: 227 calories, 29 g protein, 4.5 g carbohydrate, 9 g fat, 1.7 g saturated fat, 3.2 g monounsaturated fat, 3.4 g polyunsaturated fat, 137 mg cholesterol, .2 g fiber, 288 mg sodium. Calories from fat: 39 percent. Omega-3 fatty acids = 1.7 grams, Omega-6 fatty acids = 1.7 grams.

Salmon Cobb Salad
Makes 4 servings

8 cups (or more) coarsely chopped romaine lettuce

12 ounces cooked or grilled salmon, coarsely chopped

4 hard boiled egg whites, chopped (include two of the yolks if desired)

4 garden fresh or vine ripened tomatoes, cut into wedges

6 tablespoons bleu cheese, crumbled (optional)

6 slices crisply cooked turkey bacon, crumbled

1 avocado, peeled, pitted, and diced

1/2 cup light salad dressing of your choice (preferably with canola or olive oil)

1. Distribute shredded lettuce into 4 individual salad plates or bowls. Arrange the salmon, chopped egg, tomatoes, blue cheese, turkey bacon bits, and avocado on top of the lettuce, each in its own section.

2. Drizzle about 1/8 cup of dressing over each salad and serve!

Per serving: 409 calories, 37 g protein, 18 g carbohydrate, 21 g fat, 5 g saturated fat, 10.4 g monounsaturated fat, 5.2 g polyunsaturated fat, 87 mg cholesterol, 7 g fiber, 859 mg sodium. Calories from fat: 46 percent. Omega-3 fatty acids = 1.6 grams, Omega-6 fatty acids = 3.2 grams.

Dad's Favorite Flank Steak

There's just something about marinated flank steak that looks, smells, and tastes spectacular. We have trimmed back on sodium, fat, and calories in this recipe. On top of the health benefits, a lower-fat marinade also helps decrease the amount of HCA's (heterocyclic amines which are thought to work with food fat to promote cancer growth) potentially forming and depositing on the meat.

Makes 6 servings (3 ounces of cooked steak per serving if using a 1 1/2- pound flank steak)

2 tablespoons canola oil

6 tablespoons concentrated chicken broth (lower sodium if available)

1/2 cup honey

1/2 cup lower sodium soy sauce

4 green onions (white and part of green) cut into thin, diagonal slices

1 teaspoon ground ginger (or 2 teaspoons fresh, minced ginger)

1 teaspoon garlic powder (or 2 teaspoons fresh, minced garlic)

2 teaspoons Worcestershire sauce

1 medium-large flank steak (about 1 1/2 pounds at least)

1. Combine canola oil, chicken broth, honey, soy sauce, green onions, ginger, garlic powder, and Worcestershire sauce in a medium bowl with whisk; set aside.

2. Remove any visible fat from the flank. Lightly score the meat with a serrated knife, about 1/4-inch into the meat, in a crisscross

pattern (about an inch between cuts) on the top and bottom of the flank.

3. Add flank to rectangular plastic container and add the marinade and coat the steak well all over. Cover and marinate the flank steak all day or overnight, turning occasionally.

4. Grill about 10 to15 minutes on each side or until cooked to your desired doneness. Cut diagonally across the grain of the meat with a carving knife into slices of your desired thickness.

Per serving (including half of the marinade): 232 calories, 24 g protein, 12.5 g carbohydrate, 9 g fat, 3 g saturated fat, 4.5 g monounsaturated fat, 1 g polyunsaturated fat, 57 mg cholesterol, .2 g fiber, 460 mg sodium. Calories from fat: 35 percent. Omega-3 fatty acids = .3 gram, Omega-6 fatty acids = .6 gram.

Light Irish Lamb Stew

Here's an easy recipe for lamb stew that actually tastes better the next day! Just whip up a batch of the stew, refrigerate it overnight, and reheat it the next day for eating.

Makes 8 servings

8 slices turkey bacon

3 pounds boneless lamb shoulder, trimmed of any visible fat and cut into 2-inch pieces

1/4 teaspoon ground black pepper

1/4 cup all-purpose flour

1/4 teaspoon salt

2 tablespoons canola oil, divided use

2 cloves garlic, minced

1/2 large onion, chopped

1/4 cup water

2 cups lower sodium beef broth (regular can also be used)

1 teaspoon white sugar

4 cups diced carrots (about 4 carrots)

1 large onion, cut into bite-size pieces

2 medium potatoes with skin, diced

1/2 teaspoon dried thyme

1 bay leaf

1/2 cup white wine

1. Sauté turkey bacon slices in large nonstick skillet or frying pan, let cook then crumble into small pieces.

2. Put lamb, salt, pepper, and flour in large mixing bowl. Toss to coat meat evenly.

3. Coat bottom of large, nonstick skillet or frying pan with 1 tablespoon canola oil and brown meat over medium-high heat on all sides (about 5 to 7 minutes). If you want to fry the meat in two batches, coat the pan each time with 1/2 tablespoon of the oil.

4. Put browned meat into stockpot. Add another tablespoon of canola oil to the frying pan and sauté the garlic and yellow onion until onion begins to become golden.

5. Deglaze frying pan with 1/2-cup water and add the garlic-onion mixture to the stockpot with bacon pieces, beef broth, and sugar. Cover and simmer for 1 1/2 hours or until tender.

6. Add remaining ingredients to pot and simmer covered for 30 to 35 minutes (until vegetables are tender.)

Per serving: 450 calories, 38 g protein, 26 g carbohydrate, 19 g fat, 6.4 g saturated fat, 9 g monounsaturated fat, 3.1 g polyunsaturated fat, 123 mg cholesterol, 4 g fiber, 378 mg sodium. Calories from fat: 38 percent. Omega-3 fatty acids = .7 gram, Omega-6 fatty acids = 2.3 grams.

Beef and Beer Chili
Makes 6 servings

2 teaspoons canola oil

1 pound beef top round (such as London Broil), trimmed of fat and cut into 1/4-inch cubes

1 cup finely chopped onion

2 teaspoons minced or chopped garlic

1 teaspoon paprika

2 to 3 teaspoons chili powder

1/2 teaspoon ground cumin

1 teaspoon dried oregano flakes

14.5-ounce can low sodium Mexican-style stewed tomatoes (or similar)

1 cup light or non-alcoholic beer (beef broth or water can be substituted)

1 to 2 teaspoons finely chopped chili pepper (jalapeno chili, halved and seeded (optional), finely chopped

15-ounce can low sodium kidney beans (or pinto beans) drained and rinsed

Finely minced onion for serving (optional)

Grated reduced-fat sharp cheddar or Monterey Jack cheese (optional)

1. Heat the oil over medium-high heat in a large, nonstick frying pan or skillet. Add beef, onion, and garlic, stirring occasionally, until browned (about 3 minutes).

2. Spoon beef mixture into crock pot. Add paprika, chili powder, cumin, oregano, and stewed tomatoes (including liquid), beer, jalapeno if desired, and beans. Stir to combine. Cover and turn crock pot on LOW. Cook 8 to 10 hours.

3. Sprinkle each serving with minced onion and grated cheese if desired.

Per serving: 238 calories, 23 g protein, 23 g carbohydrate, 6 g fat, 2.1 g saturated fat, 3 g monounsaturated fat, .8 g polyunsaturated fat, 25 mg cholesterol, 8 g fiber, 189 mg sodium. Calories from fat: 23 percent. Omega-3 fatty acids = .3 gram, Omega-6 fatty acids = .5 gram.

Lean Mean Bronco Burger
Makes 4 servings

4 tablespoons canned chopped Ortega peppers

1 1/2 pounds ground sirloin (around 6 percent fat)

1/2 teaspoon ground black pepper

4 tablespoons barbeque sauce (your choice of brand)

2 tablespoons minced onion

2 teaspoons Worcestershire sauce

1/2 teaspoon garlic powder

4 whole wheat or whole grain hamburger buns

4 slices reduced fat Jack cheese (pepper jack can be substituted)

1. Preheat grill (indoor or outdoor) for high heat. Add Ortega peppers, ground sirloin, black pepper, BBQ sauce, onion, Worcestershire sauce, and garlic powder to a large bowl and use your hands or a dinner fork to mix together.

2. Divide beef mixture into 4 balls then flatten into patties (about 4-inches wide and 3/4-inch thick).

Grill or pan-fry burgers for about 4 to 5 minutes per side or until done to your liking. If pan-frying, use a nonstick frying pan or skillet and coat both sides of the burger lightly with canola cooking spray.

4. Remove burgers from the grill or frying pan to serving plate and top immediately with desired cheese.

5. Place buns on grill or in toaster oven to toast if desired.

6. Assemble burger by adding the cheese topped burgers to the toasted buns. Enjoy!

Per serving: 419 calories, 42 g protein, 30 g carbohydrate, 14.5 g fat, 6.5 g saturated fat, 5 g monounsaturated fat, 1.5 g polyunsaturated fat, 90 mg cholesterol, 4 g fiber, 637 mg sodium. Calories from fat, 31 percent. Omega-3 fatty acids = .1 gram, Omega-6 fatty acids = 1.3 grams.

Veggie Calzone

This recipe calls for a bread machine to make the calzone dough, but you can also do it by hand—just add the dough ingredients to a large bowl, mix, and then knead mixture for 15 minutes. While the bread machine is kneading the dough, you can lightly cook the broccoli and start pan-frying the eggplant.

Makes 4 servings

1 cup shredded, part-skim mozzarella cheese

1/4 cup reduced-fat goat cheese, coarsely chopped

1/4 cup shredded Parmesan cheese

1/2 regular eggplant or 1 Japanese eggplant

1 1/2 cups chopped broccoli florets, lightly cooked in microwave or steamer

1-cup fresh basil leaves

1 tablespoon olive oil

Dash red pepper flakes (optional)

1/2 teaspoon crumbled dried basil

Dough:

1 1/8 cups lukewarm water

1 tablespoon olive oil

2 tablespoons sugar

1 1/2 cups bread flour or unbleached white flour (plus extra for rolling out the dough)

1 1/2 cups whole wheat pastry flour

1 teaspoon salt

1 1/2 teaspoons rapid rise or bread machine yeast

1. For calzone dough, place water, oil, sugar, flours, salt, and yeast in bread machine pan in the order recommended by the manufacturer. Set bread machine to DOUGH cycle and press START.

2. Let the bread machine complete the mixing and kneading cycle (about 15 minutes). Remove dough from pan. Let rest on lightly floured surface for 15 minutes. Divide into 4 portions and let rest 10 minutes more.

3. While calzone dough is mixing in the bread machine, cut eggplant into 1/4-inch-wide round slices.

4. Heat a large nonstick frying pan over medium heat. Generously coat the pan with canola cooking spray. Cover bottom of pan with eggplant slices. Spray tops with canola cooking spray.

When bottoms are lightly browned (about 3 minutes) flip over and brown other side (3 minutes more). Remove from pan to cool.

5. Preheat oven to 450 degrees. Roll each portion of dough into a circle, and then stretch it into a circle 8- to 10-inches in diameter.

6. Sprinkle half of the mozzarella and all of the goat cheese, Parmesan cheese, eggplant slices, fresh basil leaves, and broccoli over half of all four of the dough circles (to make a semi-circle). Top with remaining mozzarella cheese.

7. Fold dough over to form a half circle. Moisten edges with water and then crimp the edges together. Place calzones on a cookie sheet.

8. Combine 1 tablespoon olive oil with red pepper flakes. Brush top surface of dough with olive oil mixture. Bake for 15 to 20 minutes or until calzone becomes crisp underneath and golden brown on top.

Per serving: 550 calories, 27 g protein, 76 g carbohydrate, 15 g fat, 6.6 g saturated fat, 7 g monounsaturated fat, 1.3 g polyunsaturated fat, 28 mg cholesterol, 9 g fiber, 800 mg sodium. Calories from fat: 25 percent. Omega-3 fatty acids = .1 gram, Omega-6 fatty acids = 1.1 grams.

Light Mediterranean Pasta Salad
Makes 4 servings

4 cups cooked whole wheat blend pasta or whole wheat pasta, rinsed, and drained (penne, fusilli, or farfalle shapes work well)

1/4 cup chopped bell peppers

1/4 cup chopped red onion

1/4 cup chopped sundried tomato (drained if from a jar)

1/2 cup chopped artichoke hearts, from frozen (drained if from a jar or can)

2 tablespoons sliced pitted kalamata olives

1 tablespoon capers, drained

Dressing:

2 tablespoons extra virgin olive oil

1 1/2 tablespoons champagne or red wine vinegar

1 1/2 tablespoons balsamic vinegar

1/4 teaspoon salt

1/4 teaspoon ground pepper (add more to taste if desired)

1/4 cup finely chopped fresh basil

1 tablespoon finely chopped fresh parsley

Garnish (optional):

1 tablespoon chopped sun-dried tomato (drained if from a jar)

1/4 cup fat free or light sour cream or Greek plain yogurt

1. In large serving bowl, combine salad ingredients (pasta, bell peppers, red onion, sun-dried tomato, artichoke hearts, olives and capers.)

2. In a small bowl, combine dressing ingredients with whisk.

3. Drizzle dressing over the pasta salad and toss to blend. Serve immediately or keep covered in refrigerator until ready to serve.

4. For an optional garnish, in a small food processor, combine a tablespoon of chopped sun-dried tomatoes with 1/4 cup of sour cream or Greek yogurt. Garnish each serving with a small dollop if desired.

Per serving: 282 calories, 9 g protein, 44 g carbohydrate, 8 g fat, 1 g saturated fat, 6 g monounsaturated fat, 1.1 g polyunsaturated fat, 0 mg cholesterol, 6 g fiber, 440 mg sodium. Calories from fat: 25 percent. Omega-3 fatty acids = .1 g, Omega-6 fatty acids = 1 g.

Toasted Almond Tofu Pattie Melts

If you like tofu, you will love this burger. And if you've never tried tofu, you might actually like this new dish. A serving of this vegetarian burger contributes a few vital food ingredients that help lower our serum lipid levels: soy, almonds, and flaxseed.

Makes 4 patty melts

1/2 cup grated carrot

1/2 cup thinly sliced green onions

2 teaspoons minced ginger

1 teaspoon minced or chopped garlic

12 ounces firm tofu, drained, patted dry and crumbled (about 2 cups)

1/2 cup finely chopped roasted almonds (lightly salted or unsalted both work)

4 teaspoons light or lower sodium soy sauce

1 teaspoon sesame oil

2 tablespoons ground flaxseed

2 large egg whites

2 whole grain buns, toasted (or 4 slices of whole wheat bread, toasted)

4 tomato slices

About 1/2 cup reduced-fat shredded cheese (sharp cheddar, Jack, etc.)

1. Coat a medium nonstick skillet with canola cooking spray and heat over medium heat. Add grated carrot, green onions, ginger, and garlic. Sauté until slightly softened, about 3 minutes.

2. Mix carrot mixture, tofu, almonds, soy sauce, sesame oil, and flaxseed together in a medium sized bowl with a pastry blender or fork.

3. Add egg whites to a small mixing bowl and beat on medium speed until foamy. Stir egg whites into the carrot tofu mixture.

4. Add 1/2 cup of mixture to a plastic patty press (or use palms of your hands) to form a patty about 4 1/2 inches in diameter. Repeat with the remaining mixture to make 4 patties.

5. Heat a large, nonstick frying pan or skillet with canola cooking spray over medium heat. Add patties and cook until bottom is nicely browned (about 3 to 4 minutes). Flip patties over to brown other side (about 3 to 4 minutes more).

Add one patty to each bun half. Top each patty with a tomato slice. Sprinkle 1/8 cup of shredded cheese over each patty and broil, 6 inches away from the flame or heat, until cheese melts (about a minute or two).

Per serving: 324 calories, 21 g protein, 28 g carbohydrate, 14 g fat, 3 g saturated fat, 7 g monounsaturated fat, 4 g polyunsaturated fat, 8 mg cholesterol, 7 g fiber, 474 mg sodium. Calories from fat: 39 percent. Omega-3 fatty acids = .4 gram, Omega-6 fatty acids = 3 grams.

Tofu Lasagna

The tofu replaces the ricotta cheese in this lasagna recipe. You can add some helpful veggies too (try chopped spinach from frozen, thinly sliced zucchini, grated carrot, finely diced eggplant, or any other veggie that sounds good). This recipe makes an 8 x 8-inch lasagna, but if you want a 9 x 13-inch lasagna, just double all of the ingredients.

Makes 4 servings

2 cups low sodium bottled marinara sauce, divided use

6 whole grain lasagna noodles, boiled and drained

9 ounces firm tofu crumbled (about 1 3/4 cup)

1 large egg (higher omega-3 egg if available)

1/8 teaspoon black pepper

1/8 teaspoon ground nutmeg

1 teaspoon oregano flakes

1 1/2 cup shredded part-skim mozzarella cheese, divided use

1 1/2 cups raw veggie of choice (chopped spinach from frozen or thinly sliced zucchini, grated carrot, or diced eggplant)

1/4 cup shredded Parmesan cheese

1. Preheat oven to 350 degrees. Coat an 8 x 8-inch baking dish with canola cooking spray.

2. Spread 1/2 cup of the marinara sauce in the bottom of the baking dish. Lay two of the noodles on top, breaking them apart so they fit.

3. In medium bowl, combine crumbled tofu, egg, pepper, nutmeg, 1 cup of the marinara, oregano, and 1 cup of the mozzarella

cheese. Spread half of this mixture on top of the noodles in the dish. Top with half of your veggies.

4. Cover the veggies with two more noodles then spread the remaining tofu mixture on top of the noodles followed by the remainder of the veggies.

5. Cover the veggies with the last two noodles and spread the remaining 1/2 cup of marinara on top. Sprinkle with the remaining mozzarella followed by the Parmesan cheese.

6. Bake for about 35 minutes or until top is lightly brown.

Per serving: 420 calories, 29 g protein, 53 g carbohydrate, 10.5 g fat, 5 g saturated fat, 3.5 g monounsaturated fat, 2 g polyunsaturated fat, 78 mg cholesterol, 8 g fiber, 418 mg sodium, calories from fat: 22 percent. Omega-3 fatty acids = .3 gram, Omega-6 fatty acids = 1.3 grams.

Desserts

Fresh Fruit Ice Cream Sundae

This sundae is a healthful option for hot fudge sundae lovers. Make your ice cream dessert this way and you are getting 2 grams of fiber along with a nice dose of the antioxidant vitamins like vitamin C and key minerals like calcium and potassium.

Makes 1 serving

1/2 cup light vanilla ice cream

1/2 cup assorted fresh or frozen fruit (like diced honeydew melon, sliced strawberries, and blueberries)

1 to 2 pinches ground cinnamon

1/2 teaspoon honey

1. Using a cookie dough scoop, make two to three mini scoops of ice cream and place in serving bowl (about 1/2 cup total of ice cream).

2. Top with assorted fresh or frozen fruit. Sprinkle a pinch or two of ground cinnamon over the top then drizzle some honey over the top. Enjoy!

Per serving: 151 calories, 4 g protein, 27.5 g carbohydrate, 3.5 g fat, 2 g saturated fat, 1 g monounsaturated fat, .3 g polyunsaturated fat, 18 mg cholesterol, 2 g fiber, 55 mg sodium. Calories from fat: 21 percent. Omega-3 fatty acids = .1 gram, Omega-6 fatty acids = .2 gram.

Apple Pie Crisp

Most Americans love apple pie. Well, this is the lower calorie version—Apple Pie Crisp. With the wonderful crumb topping, you will hardly notice there isn't any pie crust.

Makes 8 servings

Crisp Topping:

1/2 cup walnuts

1/2 cup unbleached white flour

1/2 cup whole wheat flour

3 tablespoons brown sugar

1/4 teaspoon ground cinnamon

3 tablespoons no trans, margarine with 8 grams fat per tablespoon, melted (in microwave or small saucepan)

3 tablespoons maple syrup, pancake syrup, or lite pancake syrup

Filling:

4 cups cored and thinly sliced apples (Pippin and Granny Smith work great), firmly packed

1/4 cup sugar (2 tablespoons Splenda can be substituted for 2 tablespoons of the sugar)

1 teaspoon apple pie spice

2 tablespoons unbleached flour

1. Preheat oven to 375-degrees. Coat a 9 x 9-inch baking dish or 9-inch cake pan or deep-dish pie plate with canola cooking spray.

2. Toast the walnuts by spreading on a pie plate and heating in oven until fragrant (about 7 minutes). Chop the nuts medium-fine.

3. Combine the flours, brown sugar, and cinnamon in a mixing bowl. Drizzle the melted margarine and maple syrup over the top and blend on LOW speed until crumbly.

4. Add the chopped nuts and mix well. The topping can be prepared up to a week ahead and refrigerated.

5. Put the sliced apples in a large bowl. Add the sugar and apple pie spice to a 1-cup measure then pour over the apples and toss. Sprinkle the 2 tablespoons flour over the apples and mix gently. Pour the mixture evenly into the prepared baking dish.

6. Spoon the topping over the apples, pressing down lightly. Place the dish on a baking sheet (if necessary) to catch any overflow. Bake on the center rack of oven until the topping is golden brown and the juices have thickened slightly, about 35-45 minutes.

7. Serve warm with light vanilla ice cream, if desired.

Per serving: 227 Calories, 4 g protein, 37 g carbohydrate, 7.5 g fat (.7 g saturated fat, 2.7 g monounsaturated fat, 3.8 g polyunsaturated fat), 0 mg cholesterol, 3 g fiber, 35 mg sodium. Calories from fat: 35 percent. Omega-3 fatty acids = 1 gram, Omega-6 fatty acids = 4 grams.

Chewy Dark Chocolate Chip Oatmeal Cookies
Makes 22 large cookies

1/2 cup light margarine with plant sterols (like Smart Balance Heart Right Light)

1/2 cup brown sugar, packed

1/4 cup white sugar (Splenda can be substituted)

1/4 cup egg substitute

6 tablespoons each of white and whole wheat flour (or 3/4 cup whole wheat flour)

1/2 teaspoon baking soda

1/2 teaspoon salt

1 teaspoon pure vanilla extract

1 cup bittersweet or semi-sweet chocolate chips

1 cup quick-cooking oatmeal

1/2 cup chopped pecans or walnuts (optional)

1.   Preheat oven to 375 degrees.

2.   In mixing bowl, combine butter, cream cheese, brown and white sugars. Add egg substitute and beat well.

3.   Add flour, baking soda, salt, and vanilla to butter mixture and beat until well blended. Stir in chocolate chips, oatmeal, and nuts if desired. Blend thoroughly.

4.   Use a cookie scoop to drop cookie dough onto a cookie sheet coated with canola cooking spray. You can spray the bottom of a flat-bottomed glass with canola cooking spray and press the cookie dough balls to make a flatter cookie.

Bake in center of oven until lightly golden (about 8 minutes). Remove cookies and let cool on wire rack.

Per serving (1 cookie): 135 calories, 4 g protein, 20 g carbohydrate, 4.5 g fat, 2 g saturated fat, 1 g monounsaturated fat, 1 g polyunsaturated fat, 12 mg cholesterol, 2 g fiber 198 mg sodium. Calories from fat: 29 percent. Omega-3 fatty acids = .2 gram, Omega-6 fatty acids = .6 gram.

Oat Berry Bars

Use the margarine cold from the refrigerator, as it will crumble more easily. Each bar contributes 1.4 grams of plant sterols as well.

Makes 24 bars

2 cups old-fashioned rolled oats

1 cup whole wheat flour

1 cup unbleached white flour

3/4 cup dark brown sugar, packed

3/4 teaspoon baking soda

3/4 teaspoon salt

1 1/4 cup light margarine with plant sterols (i.e. Smart Balance Heart Right Light with 5 grams fat and 1.7 grams plant sterols per tablespoon)

1 1/2 cups low sugar berry preserves (i.e. Smuckers Low Sugar Strawberry Preserves)

1. Preheat oven to 350 degrees. Coat a 9 x 13-inch baking dish with canola cooking spray.

2. In large mixing bowl, combine oats, whole wheat and white flours, brown sugar, baking soda, and salt by beating on low speed.

Add the margarine to the oat mixture, cold from the refrigerator, breaking it up into small pieces with your fingers or two knives or forks. Run mixer on low speed just until a crumbly mixture forms.

3. Press half of the oat mixture onto bottom of prepared baking dish. Bake until just set (about 15 minutes). Spread berry preserves evenly over warm bottom crust. Sprinkle the remaining crumb mixture evenly over the top, breaking it up into smaller pieces with fingers if necessary.

4. Bake 15 minutes more. Let cool in pan before cutting into 24 squares.

Per serving: 170 calories, 4 g protein, 28 g carbohydrate, 5 g fat, 1.4 g saturated fat, 1.6 g monounsaturated fat, 1.7 g polyunsaturated fat, 0 mg cholesterol, 3 g fiber, 180 mg sodium. Calories from fat: 25 percent. Omega-3 fatty acids = .22 gram, Omega-6 fatty acids = 1.5 grams.

Better-For-You Brownies
Makes 16 brownies

3/4 cup bittersweet chocolate chips

1/4 cup canola oil

1/4 cup fat-free sour cream

2 large eggs (high omega-3 if available)

2 tablespoons egg substitute

1 1/3 cup powdered sugar

1/3 cup granulated sugar

2 teaspoons vanilla extract

1/2 teaspoon salt

3/4 cup whole wheat flour

1/2 teaspoon baking powder

1 cup toasted pecan pieces (walnuts can be substituted)

1. Preheat oven to 350 degrees. Coat an 8 x 8-inch baking dish with canola cooking spray.

2. Combine chocolate chips and canola oil in microwave-safe glass measure or similar and microwave on HIGH for 1 minute. Stir with fork to combine and finish melting the chocolate chips. Stir in the sour cream and set aside.

3. In large mixing bowl, on medium speed, beat together eggs, egg substitute, sugars, and vanilla using an electric mixer with a paddle attachment for about 5 minutes. With mixer on low speed, beat in the melted chocolate.

4. In small bowl, combine salt, whole wheat flour, and baking powder with fork. With mixer on low speed, add the flour mixture and beat just until combined. Gently fold in the nuts.

5. Pour batter into the prepared baking dish and bake in center of oven until almost set (about 30 minutes). A toothpick inserted in the center will be slightly moist. Remove and cool slightly before serving.

Per serving (1 brownie): 202 calories, 3 g protein, 24.5 g carbohydrate, 10 g fat, 2 g saturated fat, 5.5 g monounsaturated fat, 2.5 g polyunsaturated fat, 37 mg cholesterol, 2.5 g fiber, 110 mg sodium. Calories from fat: 45 percent. Omega-3 fatty acids = .5 gram, Omega-6 fatty acids = 2 grams.

Best Berry Buckle
Makes 9 servings

1/2 cup light margarine with plant sterols added (such as Smart Balance Heart Right Light)

3/4 cup brown sugar

2 large eggs (higher omega-3 if available)

1/4 cup egg substitute

2 teaspoons vanilla extract

1/2 cup whole wheat flour

1/2 cup unbleached white flour

1/2 teaspoon salt

1/2 teaspoon baking powder

1 teaspoon ground cinnamon

3 cups raspberries or mixed berries

Powdered sugar, for dusting (optional)

1. Preheat oven to 350 degrees. Coat a 9 x 9-inch bakind dish with canola cooking spray.

2. In large mixing bowl, combine margarine and brown sugar with electric mixer until fluffy and well blended. Add eggs and egg substitute, one at a time, beating after each addition. Add vanilla and beat until blended.

3. In medium bowl, combine flours, salt, baking powder, and cinnamon with whisk. On low speed, gradually add flour mixture to egg batter, beating just until blended. Scrape sides of bowl with spatula and make sure and stir everything together.

4. Spread batter in prepared baking dish. Scatter berries evenly on top and gently press down a bit to sink some of the raspberries. Bake until toothpick inserted in center comes out clean and top is golden brown (about 45 minutes).

5. Let cool 20 minutes. Dust with powdered sugar if desired.

Per serving: 198 calories, 4.5 g protein, 33 g carbohydrate, 6 g fat, .8 g saturated fat, 2.2 g monounsaturated fat, 2 g polyunsaturated fat, 52 mg cholesterol, 4 g fiber, 274 mg sodium. Calories from fat: 24 percent. Omega-3 fatty acids = .2 gram, Omega-6 fatty acids = 1.6 grams.

Chapter 5

Take the Heart Smart Supermarket Tour

Wouldn't it be awesome if you could sign up at your local supermarket and take a one-hour tour with a dietitian who would point out all the things you need to know, aisle by aisle, to eat heart smart? Well, some innovative supermarkets offer such a thing, but most don't. So take this virtual tour with me as your guide. You don't have to write down any notes (they are already written down here)…and the best part is you can take the tour whenever it's convenient for you! Let's start with a label lesson.

Foods to Keep Out of Your Shopping Cart

Watch out for the three-S's while reading the labels on those food packages: sugar, saturated fat (and trans fat), and sodium. These are the three nutrients that people in the U.S. get too much of. Fortunately, all three can be found on the Nutrition Facts label of packaged foods.

How do you make sure you aren't getting too much of these three? Buy processed food and fast food a lot less often and, when you do put them in the shopping cart, check the label, and make sure you are buying options that are lower in sugar, saturated fat, and sodium.

There are four main things to look for on the food label.

1. Understanding Carbohydrates

Have you looked at a Nutrition Facts label lately? In bold you will easily find "total carbohydrate," but on many product labels there are all sorts of different carbohydrate terms listed underneath that such as dietary fiber, sugar, other carbohydrates, and sometimes sugar alcohols. That's enough to confuse any of us!

On The Label: Total Carbohydrate

If you are diabetic and you need to track your grams of carbohydrate, it's the "total carbohydrate" line that will interest you the most. "Net carbohydrates," a term often used in low carbohydrate diets, refers to the total amount of carbohydrate (in grams) minus the grams of dietary fiber. You'll find that often the grams of fiber, grams of sugars, and grams of other carbohydrate will add up to the grams of total carbohydrate on the label.

On The Label: Dietary Fiber

This is the total amount of fiber in the product, which means this is the amount of carbohydrate that is indigestible and will likely pass through the intestinal tract without being absorbed. Fiber keeps things running right in the intestines, reduces the risk of coronary heart disease, and assists in keeping blood sugar levels normal, according to the Dietary Reference Intakes report.

The guideline: get about 30 grams of total fiber a day from a variety of foods. Fiber is found in plant foods, pure and simple. Follow these foods and you'll find some fiber:

- All vegetables (fresh, frozen, and canned)
- All fruits (fresh, frozen, and canned)

- All types of beans (dried, canned, fresh)
- Edamame (fresh or frozen) and other soybean products
- Nuts and seeds
- Whole grains and whole grain cereal (hot and cold)
- 100% whole wheat or whole grain bread, buns, pitas, rolls, tortillas
- Whole grain blend pastas
- Whole grain crackers

On The Label: Sugars

"Sugars" is also listed on the Nutrition Facts label and this number includes ALL sugars--including natural sources like milk sugars (lactose) and the fructose and glucose from fruits and dried fruits. Your average 1% low-fat milk label will list 15 grams of "sugar" per cup. Those grams are from the lactose (milk sugars), not any sweetener that has been added to the milk. If you want to get an idea of how much of the sugars on the label are from added sugars like high fructose corn syrup or white or brown sugar, check the list of ingredients on the label and see if any of those sweeteners are in the top three or four ingredients. The Nutrition Facts label for Kellogg's Raisin Bran lists 19 grams of "sugars" per cup, but if you check the ingredient list, you find that the first three ingredients are whole wheat, raisins, and wheat bran. The fourth and fifth ingredients are sugar and high fructose corn syrup.

On The Label: Sugar Alcohols

Some product labels also break out sugar alcohols under total carbohydrate. Some people are particularly motivated to look for these because sugar alcohols can cause intestinal issues (gas, cramping, diarrhea) for some people even at low levels. If you look on the ingredient label, the sugar alcohols include terms such as sorbitol, lactitol, mannitol, and others. Keep in mind that many of the "sugar free" or "reduced-calorie" products contain some sugar alcohols even when another alternative sweetener like Splenda is in the product. For example, Sugar Free Fudgicles are sweetened with Splenda and yet a quick glance at the Nutrition Facts label shows you that each serving (2 pops) also contains 6 grams of sugar alcohol.

2. Total Fat and The Bad Fats (Saturated Fat and Trans Fat)

On The Label: Total Fat/Saturated Fat/Trans Fat (Grams)

If you are striving to meet the guideline to get 7 percent or less of your total calories from saturated fat and you eat about 2,000 calories a day, that calculates to 16 grams of saturated fat a day.

The guideline: Shoot for less than 20 grams of saturated fat a day and strive for no trans fats in the foods you buy.

Label Tip: Look for both saturated fat and trans fat on the nutrition information label on all processed and packaged foods.

3. The Smart Fats (monounsaturated fat and omega-3s)

On The Label: Monounsaturated Fat (Grams)/ Polyunsaturated Fat (Grams)

Polyunsaturated Fat represents omega-3 fatty acids and omega-6 fatty acids combined. Good choices at the supermarket include fatty fish and other fish to a lesser extent, nuts (such as walnuts and almonds), seeds such as ground flaxseed, olive, and canola oil and products made with them, and higher omega-3 eggs.

4. Sodium Can Add Up Quickly in Processed and Packaged Food

On The Label: Sodium (Milligrams)

The foods most likely to be high in sodium are the snack foods and other processed foods, frozen snack foods and frozen dinners, cold cuts, and packaged meats. Fresh fruits and vegetables and fresh meats obviously don't have a label that tells you the sodium content, but it's naturally low in these foods anyway!

The guideline: shoot for less than 2,000 milligrams of sodium a day for adults (your doctor might even suggest less than 1,500 milligrams for some of you).

The Supermarket Tour

It's easy to get lost in the details when you are walking through the supermarket, but I want to give you some general advice. The best way to get more of the nutrients you need and less of those that contribute to disease and extra calories is to simply serve more whole foods and less processed food. One of the best ways to do this is to cook homemade meals more often and to reach for foods that don't even come with a nutrition label such as broccoli, spinach, apples, grapes, avocados, brown rice, whole wheat flour, salmon, chicken breast, almonds, kidney beans, or olive oil.

The Bread Aisle: Make the switch to whole grain breads

Every time you eat a slice of bread—as toast, part of a sandwich, or an ingredient in a recipe—you've got an opportunity to improve your diet by switching to whole grains.

Many people have a sandwich almost every day; there's two slices of whole grain right there. Some of us enjoy toast, bagels, or English muffins with breakfast; 100 percent whole-wheat options are now available. When you make yourself a grilled chicken sandwich, hamburger, or hot dog, you can add two more servings of whole grain by buying 100 percent whole-wheat buns.

Whole grains are naturally low in fat and cholesterol-free, contain 10 to 15 percent protein, and offer loads of fiber, resistant starch, minerals, vitamins, antioxidants, phytochemicals, and often, phytoestrogens. With all those nutrients in one package, it's no wonder whole grains provide so many health benefits, including protection from cardiovascular disease, stroke, diabetes, insulin resistance, obesity, and some cancers.

Two bread myths busted

MYTH: If it's brown and has the word "wheat" in the name, it has lots of fiber and is 100 percent whole grain.

TRUTH: The first ingredient listed on the ingredient label tells the story. If its "wheat flour" or "enriched bleached flour" (or similar), that tells you white flour was mostly used, not "whole wheat" flour.

MYTH: Bread with healthy sounding names like "seven-grain" or "100 percent natural" are nutrition stars.

TRUTH: Look beyond the name. Just because the name of the bread on the package sounds healthy, doesn't mean it is. Oroweat's 7-grain and 12-grain bread, for example, list "unbleached enriched flour" as the first ingredient. Nature's Pride 100% Natural Honey Wheat bread, likewise, is mainly made with "wheat flour."

Top bread choices in chain supermarkets

All of the following bread products have:

- 4 grams of fiber per 2-slice serving (or similar)
- 100 percent whole-wheat flour as the first ingredient
- Less than 401 mg sodium per 2-slice serving
- 1 gram saturated fat or less per 2-slice serving (but most have zero saturated fat)

English Muffins (1 whole)	Calories	Fiber	Sodium	Carbs	Protein
Oroweat Whole Grain & Flax (64 g) (Contains whole flax-seed and Menhaden oil—fish oil for a total of 14 mg of EPA/DHA omega-3s)	150	5	160	29	5
Oroweat 100% whole wheat (59 g)	130	4	240	25	5
Bagel & Buns (1 whole)	Calories	Fiber	Sodium	Carbs	Protein
Oroweat Whole Grain 100% Whole Wheat Hamburger Bun (71 g)	180	6	350	31	8

Oroweat Whole Grain 100% Whole Wheat Hotdog Bun (56 g)	160	6	320	28	8
Thomas Hearty Grains 100% Whole Wheat Bagels (95 g)	240	7	400	49	10
Pita Pockets (1 whole)	Calories	Fiber	Sodium	Carbs	Protein
Thomas Sahara Pita Pockets 100% Whole Wheat (57 g)	140	4	320	28	6
Toufayan Multi-grain Pita (69 g)	173	4	288	35	8
Sliced Bread (2 slices)	Calories	Fiber	Sodium	Carbs	Protein
Milton's Whole Grain Plus Bread (76 g)	180	10	250	32	8

Oroweat Country 100% Whole Wheat (76 g)	200	6	360	36	8
Oroweat Protein Health (86 g)	200	6	360	36	12
Sara Lee Hearty & Delicious 100% Multi-grain (86 g)	240	6	400	42	10
Nature's Pride 100% Whole Wheat (56 g)	140	4	2230	26	6

The Dairy and Egg Aisle

Some people are big milk drinkers and some people aren't. I'm a lifetime member of the latter group. Nothing against milk, I just don't enjoy drinking it all by itself. I'm big on iced nonfat lattes though. But just in case you are a milk drinker, the lower-fat milks are the way to go, particularly if you have heart disease.

The fastest way to decrease calories, cholesterol, and saturated fat grams is to decrease the fat in the milk. Nonfat milk and 1% milk fat are your best health options.

Think of the savings per week or month just by switching from whole milk or 2% milk to 1% milk or nonfat. It does add up. If you drink 2 glasses of milk a day (16 ounces total), this is what you will save:

Per week:

	Saturated Fat (g)	Fat (g)	Cholesterol (mg)	Calories
Switch from whole milk to 1%milk	43	78	170	615
Switch from 2% milk to nonfat milk	38	59	205	440

Per month:

	Saturated Fat (g)	Fat (g)	Cholesterol (mg)	Calories
Switch from whole milk to 1% milk	172	312	680	2460
Switch from 2% milk to nonfat milk	152	236	820	1760

Would The Best Butter Substitute Please Stand Up?

What's better for your health, butter or margarine? I get this question a lot. The cast of characters keeps changing, too. A few years back, margarines with plant sterols added were the new kids on the butter block. Since then, there's been a mad dash to eliminate or nearly eliminate trans fats, and in the months to come, probiotics will likely be making their way into a margarine tub near you.

When it comes to the types of fat in margarine, here are a few things to keep in mind:

Monounsaturated fat is a smarter fat for your heart health and the two oils that give us the most monounsaturated fat are olive oil and canola oil.

For polyunsaturated fat, we generally don't get enough omega-3s and we get too much omega-6s in our typical American diet, but unfortunately most companies don't list the grams of each on the label. You will see the total amount of polyunsaturated fat grams and this is comprised of omega-6s and omega-3s.

Canola oil gives us some omega-3 fatty acids though; so liquid canola oil is always a good ingredient to find on a margarine label. Flaxseed oil and fish oil would also contribute omega-3s if they were added to the margarine. Soybean oil does contain some omega-3s, but it's also fairly high in omega-6s. Vegetable oils like corn oil, soybean oil, and grapeseed oil contribute the most omega-6s.

Ranking the Margarines by Flavor

Choosing a margarine that you like to use on your table and in your cooking is a big decision. Some of this is subjective of course, but I thought I would taste test the major players in the margarine section and rank them by taste. If your doctor has encouraged you to switch to the margarines with plant sterols, there are about three brands out there right now. Check out my comments on those particular margarines below and try them one at a time until you find the one that appeals to you the most.

1. Country Crock Spreadable Butter (with canola oil). The good news with this choice is it contains butter and the bad news is it contains butter. It tastes like butter because butter is the first ingredient, but the bad news is it contains more saturated fat (because of the butter).

Bottom line (taste)—It tastes great and works well in recipes. The texture is very soft (partly because it contains buttermilk and water) so you just have to keep it in the refrigerator at all times.

Bottom line (nutrition)—It has a high amount of monounsaturated fat because canola oil is the second ingredient, but it contains a stiff amount of saturated fat—3.5 grams per tablespoon.

1 tablespoon = 9 grams fat, 3.5 grams saturated fat, 0 trans fat, 1.5 grams polyunsaturated fat, 4 grams monounsaturated fat.

List of ingredients (in order of most to least): butter, canola oil, buttermilk, water

2. Land O Lakes Fresh Buttery Taste Spread. This margarine comes in BIG tubs, which can be quite economical, especially if you are planning to do a lot of baking.

Bottom line (taste)—It tastes pretty good and works well in most recipes. It's definitely margarine, but has a pleasant buttery flavor.

Bottom line (nutrition)—It contains 8 grams of fat per tablespoon, which is less than stick margarine or butter, which has about 12 grams per tablespoon. Wish it were made with canola oil instead of soybean oil so there would be more plant omega-3s, and it does contain partially hydrogenated and hydrogenated soybean oil in the ingredient list, but they are listed after (and added in smaller amounts than) liquid soybean oil and water.

1 tablespoon = 8 grams fat, 2 grams saturated fat, 0 trans fat (because this product contains partially hydrogenated oil, this "0" trans is probably

truly somewhere between .5 gram trans and zero), 3.5 grams polyunsaturated fat, 1.5 grams monounsaturated fat.

3. Brummel & Brown Spread. Yogurt is the third ingredient. Bet you didn't expect that in your margarine. I really like the look and taste of this margarine for table use. It may not work quite as well in heated or bakery recipes because it has a lot less fat per tablespoon than regular butter and the first ingredient listed is water, whereas only about 20 percent of butter is water.

Bottom line (taste)—This margarine has a nice white color and a fluffy, soft texture. It has a pleasant, mild flavor with a hint of sweetness.

Bottom line (nutrition)—It is a lot lower in fat per tablespoon than butter and most margarine. It contains a gram of saturated fat per tablespoon. Half of the fat (2.5 grams) comes from polyunsaturated fat, a small amount of which is omega-3s because the two oils used contain some omega-3s (canola oil and soybean oil).

1 tablespoon = 5 grams fat, 1 gram saturated fat, 0 trans (because this product contains partially hydrogenated oil, this "0" trans is probably truly somewhere between .5 gram and zero), 2.5 grams polyunsaturated fat, 1 gram monounsaturated fat.

4. Smart Balance Heart Right Light. This is the best-tasting margarine that contains plant sterols, in my opinion. And each tablespoon contributes a hefty dose too—1.7 grams of plant sterols.

Bottom line (taste)—This margarine has a surprisingly thick texture and a light yellow color. Although the flavor is very mild, many of my tasters found it pleasant-tasting at the same time. It may not work well in heated or bakery recipes because it has a lot less fat per tablespoon than regular butter and the first ingredient listed is water. But if you just replace exactly the butter or shortening called for (in cookies, cakes, brownies, crisps) with this light margarine, it usually will work out pretty well and you've cut the fat coming from the baking fat in half, dramatically lowered the saturated fat, and gotten your daily dose of plant sterols.

Bottom line (nutrition)—A "natural oil blend," similar to the one used to make the Smart Balance Omega Buttery Spread, is used to make this margarine, but this product has more water and therefore less fat per tablespoon than the other. This margarine also contains some omega-3s from fish and canola and soybean oil but seems to have about half as much (about .2 gram) as the Omega Buttery Spread.

1 tablespoon = 5 grams fat, 1.5 grams saturated fat, 0 trans, 1.5 grams polyunsaturated fat, 1.5 grams monounsaturated fat.

5. Smart Balance Omega Buttery Spread. I love that this margarine lists the amount of plant omega-3s (ALA) and fish omega-3s (EPA and DHA) per tablespoon.

Bottom line (taste)—This margarine has a yellowish color, light but pleasant margarine-like flavor, and a nice, stiff texture.

Bottom line (nutrition)—Although there is no hydrogenation going on in the making of this margarine, the saturated fat is 2.5 grams per tablespoon. I'm guessing, from the list of oils used in their "natural oil blend," that this is mainly coming from palm fruit oil, which contains some naturally saturated fatty acids.

The rest of the fat is pretty much split between poly-unsaturated fat and monounsaturated fat. Of the 3 grams of polyunsaturated fat per tablespoon, roughly .4 grams appears to be from omega-3s.

1 tablespoon = 8 grams fat, 2.5 grams saturated fat, 0 trans, 3 grams polyunsaturated fat, 2.5 grams monounsaturated fat.

6. **I Can't Believe It's Not Butter! Original (tub).** According to my friendly neighborhood stockperson at my grocery store, this is one of the best-selling tub margarines. I was anxious to test it and see what all the fuss was about. It wasn't altogether unappealing, but there seemed to be quite a few margarines that ranked higher in taste.

   Bottom line (taste)—Lighter color and softer texture than Smart Balance. Pleasant but margarine-like flavor.

   Bottom line (nutrition)—Until 2010, this margarine still contained hydrogenated and partially hydrogenated oil but, its parent company, Unilever, completely eliminated hydrogenated oils from its products. In 2009, a tablespoon contributed 2 grams of saturated fat and 3.5 grams of polyunsaturated (.4 grams of which are plant omega-3s from soybean and canola oil).

   1 tablespoon = 8 grams fat, 2 g saturated fat, 0 g trans, 3.5 grams polyunsaturated fat, 2 grams mono-unsaturated fat.

7. **Promise activ Light (Take Control brand) tied with Benecol Light Spread.** Water is the first ingredient in both of these products (thus the 5 grams of fat per tablespoon) so they won't act the same way in the

frying pan or in baking as other margarines. When melting in a frying pan, you might literally see the water separate out from the oil in the margarine.

Bottom line (taste)—Both of these products have a very artificial yellow color and both tasted just "okay." Benecol has a secondary subtle sweet flavor.

Bottom line (nutrition)—Both of these products contain plant sterols that help reduce serum cholesterol when consumed every day. Promise activ contains 1 gram of saturated fat per tablespoon mostly coming from two naturally saturated oils (palm oil and palm kernel oil) while Benecol contains .5 gram.

1 tablespoon (Promise) = 5 grams fat, 1 gram saturated fat, 1.5 gram polyunsaturated fat, 2.5 grams monounsaturated fat.

1 tablespoon (Benecol) = 5 grams fat, .5 gram saturated fat, 2 gram polyunsaturated fat, 2.5 grams monounsaturated fat.

When it has to be butter

There are certain bakery recipes where you are whipping sugar together with fat to create the proper texture (cakes, cookies, frosting, and so on) and you can't substitute oil. What is your best bet then? In these cases you can switch to a margarine you like. Where does that leave butter? Butter is very high in saturated fat (but not as high as the tropical oils; palm kernel and coconut oil), but contains zero trans fats, and it does contain some monounsaturated fat (but not as much as some of the vegetable oils). I've got to admit there are certain recipes where butter is the ideal cooking fat for the recipe. When butter browns it contains hundreds of flavor components and volatiles that we taste—and nothing beats that flavor. So there are some recipes that I use butter in, but I use the smallest amount I can get away with using and still have the dish taste terrific. When I can switch to canola oil, olive oil, or no trans margarine in a recipe, I do.

Canola oil or olive oil are my two favorite oils nutritionally and I'll switch to them in recipes instead of butter or shortening whenever I can. If a recipe calls for melting the butter or shortening, that's usually a good sign that you can use oil instead. I usually use a lot less, even still, than the recipe calls for.

Are Eggs Good Or Bad?

Studies are still shedding light on this very question and there are new developments in egg-laying science, too. If the feed of the chickens is changed, it changes the nutritional composition of the eggs they lay. The higher omega-3 eggs now in supermarkets across America are one example of this.

The upside of eggs is they are definitely powerhouses of key nutrients including 6 grams of high quality protein (all of which is in the egg white). Each egg yolk also contributes a nice dose of the phytochemical, lutein, thought to help ward off age-related macular degeneration (the leading cause of vision loss among older people).

The downside of eggs is that each egg yolk also contributes at least 200 milligrams of cholesterol (70 to100 percent of the recommended daily intake, depending on which guideline you use) and about 5 grams of fat, roughly 2 grams of which are saturated. And if you think about it, we never seem to eat just one egg. Most American egg dishes feature not one but two or three eggs per serving like three-egg omelets, quiches, frittatas, eggs benedict, or scrambled eggs. Consuming two or three eggs per person changes the numbers quite a bit. Now suddenly we are talking about a serving containing 15 grams of fat, 6 grams of saturated fat, and 636 milligrams of cholesterol.

For people with coronary artery disease, high cholesterol levels, or other cardiovascular risks, they may have been instructed to limit their cholesterol intake to 200 milligrams a day. A reduction in dietary cholesterol is recommended to prevent cardiovascular disease and almost everyone knows that eggs are particularly rich in cholesterol. Yet the research data published on the effect of eggs on heart disease risk has been, overall, limited and inconsistent. Also keep in mind that higher intakes of saturated fat and trans fat raise LDL (bad) cholesterol levels more than higher amounts of dietary cholesterol.

But, using data from the Physicians' Health Study I, researchers found that high egg consumption was related to a higher death rate and that this relationship was even stronger in people with diabetes. The risk of death for people who ate the highest amount of eggs per week was double what the risk of death was for people who ate the lowest amount of eggs per week. An earlier study found that among people with diabetes, consuming more than six eggs per week was associated with an increased risk of coronary artery disease.

Bottom Line: I personally am not afraid to use and enjoy eggs in my recipes and meals, I just automatically use half eggs and half egg substitute or egg white to bring down the saturated fat and cholesterol and I always purchase higher omega-3 eggs to increase the smart fats in my overall diet.

Cheese, If You Please

Yes, it's true; cheese is a source of fat, cholesterol, and, more importantly, saturated fat. The biggest contributor of saturated fat and cholesterol in the American diet is the meat group (beef, processed meats, eggs, poultry, and other meats), with the milk group as the number two contributor (also includes cream and cheese). But on the plus side, cheese is a great source of animal protein and calcium (two nutrients many of us need more of).

Just two ounces of reduced-fat cheese a day will give you about 40 to 50 percent of the daily value for calcium and around 15 grams of protein for an investment of only 160 to 180 calories (10 grams fat, 8 grams saturated fat and 20 mg cholesterol).

Two ounces of regular cheese will give you about the same amount of calcium and protein, but the calorie and fat price tag will be a bit steeper: 228 calories, 19 grams of fat, 12 grams of saturated fat, and 50 milligrams of cholesterol.

How to Be Heart Smart About Cheese

What about using cheese in recipes when you are trying to trim down and eat less fat and saturated fat?

Switch to reduced fat cheese or use half as much of regular fat cheese. The calories will decrease by 30 percent, the fat grams by about 40 percent, and the saturated fat by one-third, but the calcium and protein will still be high.

Sometimes you have to use regular cheese. There are situations certainly when a particular type of cheese is needed for the recipe and a reduced-fat version is not available—such is the case with Parmesan cheese or Gruyere. In these types of recipes, reach for the real cheese, just use less and you also might be able to cut back on fat and saturated fat in other steps and ingredients of the recipe.

Pair cheese with healthy food partners.

Because cheese is a source of saturated fat, try to pair it with lower fat and higher fiber food partners such as pears, whole wheat pasta, whole grains, beans, and even vegetables instead of high fat crackers, pastry, or high fat meats like salami or sausage.

The Cooking Oil Aisle

The simple decision of which fat we choose to cook and bake with can have a huge impact on our family's health. So which fat reigns supreme?

There are so many different nutrient issues to consider, there is really no one winner in this race. Olive oil wins by being highest in the more healthful monounsaturated fats. It doesn't contain very much plant omega-3s, however, you can't use it for high temperature frying, and it may impart an olive flavor when you bake with it. Then there's canola oil, which is lowest in saturated fat and also contains an impressive amount of monounsaturated fat (although not as high as olive oil) and contains the most omega-3 fatty acids of the vegetable oils. You can use canola oil in baking and high temperature frying, too.

The Frozen Entrée Aisle

I don't venture into this aisle often, but when I do, I'm looking for frozen entrees that don't look or taste like they're frozen entrées. You should want to enjoy that frozen entree at work or at home, again and again. I've personally had good luck with frozen entrees I've tasted at specialty type supermarkets or stores like Whole Foods and Trader Joe's. Particularly if you are looking for entrees that are organic or vegetarian, these venues may offer you several tasty options that you won't see elsewhere. But even if you are shopping in your typical supermarket, there are some choices that standout as better tasting. But are they better for you too? There's the second challenge—finding frozen entrees that taste great and are good for you.

There are three nutritional obstacles to overcome when in search for the perfect frozen entrée:

- Finding an entrée that isn't too high in sodium (hopefully less than 800 mg).
- Finding an entrée that contains enough fiber (at least 3 grams but hopefully more).
- Finding an entrée that doesn't have too much fat, particularly saturated fat (30 percent calories from fat or less unless it features a smart fat food like salmon).

Suffice it to say, some frozen entrees/dinners can get into the over 1500 milligram sodium range, some can contribute 12 to 20 grams of saturated fat alone (even more total fat), and very few offer more than three grams of fiber—the amount of fiber found in 1 medium-sized apple.

It's a good idea to have some meal items sitting in your freezer for times when you need to make something on the fly. There are some smarter carbohydrate and smarter fat choices available if you look in the right places. There are frozen grilled fish fillets in two flavors: Lemon Pepper and Garlic Butter. One fillet of either flavor contains 100 calories, 3 grams fat, .5 gram saturated fat, 60 mg cholesterol, 0 grams fiber, and 350 to 380 mg sodium.

The most popular shelf in the freezer is probably the frozen potato section. There are better options for us in this aisle, too. You can buy your frozen hash browns and shredded potato patties in the freezer section with fat already added or with zero fat. Read the label though because it's easy to mistake the ones with mega fat for the ones with no fat. When you buy them with zero fat, you can then fry them up with a little bit of canola oil or canola oil cooking spray.

For frozen french fries, you can buy options with less fat added and then bake them until crispy in the oven. Ore Ida makes several types that contain less than 4 grams of fat per 3 ounce serving such as Ore Ida Steak Fries.

The Condiment Corner

You know what I'm going to say, right? That the creamy dressings and spreads based on mayonnaise tend to be the most caloric and highest in fat grams. I'm talking about condiments such as mayonnaise, tartar sauce, and "special sauce." Sauces and spreads based on cream or sour cream are next in line, like ranch sauce. If mayo is a must, consider switching to light mayonnaise, which still adds 35 calories, 3.5 grams fat, and .5 gram saturated fat per tablespoon.

So what condiments are better for us? Anything based on a vegetable tends to be a better choice, such as salsa, ketchup, or pickle relish. The first five ingredients in my favorite salsa, for example, are tomatoes, orange juice from concentrate, tomato paste, onions, and garlic. Mustard is also a great choice, being that it's made with mainly vinegar, water, and mustard seed. Another one of my favorite condiments is barbecue sauce. One tablespoon goes a long way and adds about 30 calories, 0 grams fat, 6 grams sugar, and 120 mg sodium—depending on the brand. Barbecue sauce can also be based on tomatoes with tomato puree and tomato paste being common ingredients in most store-bought options.

- Mustard, 2 teaspoons—0 calories, 0 g fat (0 g saturated), 110 mg sodium
- Salsa, 2 tablespoons—10 calories, 0 g fat (0 g saturated), 170 mg sodium
- Bbq sauce, 1 tablespoon—30 calories, 0 g fat (0 g saturated), 120 mg sodium
- Ketchup, 1 tablespoon—15 calories, 0 g fat (0 g saturated), 190 mg sodium

The Ice Cream Aisle

Americans love their ice cream—and have ever since Thomas Jefferson brought the recipe for it home from France more than 200 years ago. The combination of sweet taste and creamy texture is in a word, magical. The good news is that you can now find most any flavor you might desire in a lower fat version. And here's even better news—many of these "light" ice cream brands taste great!

You can also find plenty of ice cream treats in which manufacturers have reduced the sugar by adding sugar alcohols. (But keep in mind that sugar alcohols can cause intestinal distress for some people—especially those with Irritable Bowel Syndrome—if they consume too much of them.)

There are five main things to look for on the label of an ice cream treat. It's not all about fat grams! Per half-cup serving (the standard serving for scoop ice cream), your best bets will have:

- 4 grams of fat or less
- around 120 calories
- 3 grams or less of saturated fat
- no more than 10 milligrams cholesterol per serving
- 15 grams of sugar or less per serving (many ice creams have almost double this amount)

The Beverage Aisle

Here's the bottom line to this aisle of the supermarket—switch from soda and fruit drinks or basically any sweetened beverages, to water, low fat milk, and unsweetened tea. If you have an abundance of healthful beverages to choose from in the kitchen (low-fat milk, iced green or black tea available in decaf, mineral water, or diet soda if you are trying to wean yourself off of regular soda), you will have an easier time avoiding the high-sugar and high-calorie drinks.

The Meat and Processed Meat Section

When it comes to eating beef and pork, the key is to buy the leaner cuts, trimming any visible fat from the meat before cooking, and cooking the meat with as little fat as possible (and using olive oil or canola oil when you do add a little fat).

Beef and Pork

What are the leaner cuts of red meat? Let your eyes tell you. The darker red the beef cut, for example, the leaner the cut. The leaner red meat choices in most supermarkets include (be sure to trim visible fat from these cuts):

- Beef and pork roasts
- Stew meat
- Round tip steak
- Top round strips

- London broil steak
- Beef tenderloin steak (filet mignon)
- Top sirloin steak
- Pork tenderloin
- Center cut pork loin chops

The more fat and marbling in the beef or ground beef, the lighter red it becomes. For some cuts and types of meat, you can literally see the ribbons or trimming of white fat. Here are a few examples of what these leaner options add up to:

- Ground beef, 7 percent fat—4 ounces raw contains 160 calories, 8 grams fat, 3 grams saturated fat, 60 mg cholesterol, and 85 mg sodium.
- London broil steak—3 ounces of broiled steak contains 176 calories, 8.5 grams fat, 3.7 grams saturated fat (3.5 g monounsaturated fat, .3 g polyunsaturated fat), and 57 mg cholesterol, 70 mg sodium.
- Beef rump roast—3 ounces of lean, braised roast contains 167 calories, 5.7 grams fat, 2 grams saturated fat (2.6 grams monounsaturated fat, .2 grams polyunsaturated fat), 81 mg cholesterol, and 43 mg sodium.
- Pork tenderloin—3 ounces of roasted tenderloin contains 140 calories, 4 grams fat, 1.4 grams saturated fat (1.6 grams monounsaturated fat, .4 gram polyunsaturated fat), and 67 mg cholesterol, 47 mg sodium.

Poultry

About half of the fat in chicken is in the skin, so obviously you are better off taking it off. Thigh meat has more fat and cholesterol than light meat, but it has a little more iron, zinc, vitamin E, and B2. Breast meat has more vitamin B3, B6, and magnesium than thigh meat.

When it comes to ground turkey or chicken, you need to check the label. You want to find products that have the same amount of fat or less than ground beef with 7 percent fat. Here are some poultry comparisons for you.

- Foster Farms Ground Turkey Lean—4 ounces raw contains 150 calories, 7 grams fat, 2 grams saturated fat, 65 mg cholesterol, and 80 mg sodium.

- Chicken breast, without skin, roasted—3 ounces contains 142 calories, 3.1 grams fat, .9 gram saturated fat (1.1 grams monounsaturated fat, .7 gram polyunsaturated fat), 73 mg cholesterol, and 63 mg sodium.

- Chicken thigh, without skin, roasted—3 ounces contains 180 calories, 9.4 grams fat, 2.6 grams saturated fat (3.6 grams monounsaturated fat, 2.1 grams polyunsaturated fat), 82 mg cholesterol, and 76 mg sodium.

The Deli Drawer

The sodium is going to be pretty high in processed meats, but you can find some leaner choices like turkey and chicken breast and lean ham. For lunchmeats, you want to look for 97 percent fat free on the label—which will generally get you to the better choices. For the higher fat deli meats, like salami and pepperoni, you'll find some 60 percent less fat choices.

- Hillshire Farm deli select honey ham—2 ounces contains 60 calories, 1.5 grams fat, .5 gram saturated fat, 25 mg cholesterol, and 500 mg sodium.

- Gallo light salami 50 percent less fat—5 slices contains 60 calories, 4 grams fat, 1.5 grams saturated fat, 25 mg cholesterol, and 520 mg sodium.

- Hormel 70 percent less fat—17 slices contains 80 calories, 4 grams fat, 1.5 grams saturated fat, 40 mg cholesterol, and 600 mg sodium.

The sodium is also going to be high in hot dogs and franks, but look out for the products with less grams of fat and saturated fat and the ones with antioxidants added (vitamin C or E as ascorbic acid, ascorbate or tocopherol or P-coumaric and chlorogenic acids) in the ingredient list. They help stop the formation of nitrosamines, which are known to have carcinogenic activity and are formed during the breakdown of the processed meat additives—nitrates and nitrites. Here are a few of the light hot dog choices out there.

- Oscar Mayer Louis Rich 1/3 less fat turkey franks—1 frank (45 grams) contains 100 calories, 8 g fat, 2.5 g saturated fat, 30 mg cholesterol, and 510 mg sodium.

- Ball Park lite franks—1 frank (50 grams) contains 100 calories, 7 g fat, 2.5 g saturated fat, 25 mg cholesterol, and 460 mg sodium.

When it comes to sausage and links, you need to find the balance between products that add enough fat that they still look and taste like sausage, but have cut out the extra fat that's really not needed. You'll find quite a few selections.

- Hillshire Farms turkey polska kielbasa—2 ounce serving contains 90 calories, 5 grams fat, 2 grams saturated fat, 35 mg cholesterol, and 540 mg sodium.

- Healthy Choice polska kielbasa or low-fat smoked sausage—2 ounce serving of either contains 80 calories, 2.5 grams fat, 1 gram saturated fat, 25 mg cholesterol, and 480 mg sodium.

- Jimmy Dean Turkey Sausage Links—3 cooked links contain 120 calories, 7 g fat, 2 g saturated fat, 55 mg cholesterol and 490 mg sodium.

- Jenni-O Sweet Italian Turkey Sausage—1 large link contains 160 calories, 10 grams fat, 2.5 grams saturated fat, 60 mg cholesterol, and 670 mg sodium.

Bacon, quite simply, is mostly pork fat. All you have to do is fry some and you'll be left with a pan full of grease. So, our only choice if you want pork bacon is to choose center cut bacon, which contains 25 to 30 percent less fat than typical bacon, or to choose some of the better turkey bacons such as Louis Rich turkey bacon (1 slice contains 35 calories, 2.5 grams fat, 1 gram saturated fat, 15 mg cholesterol, and 180 mg sodium).

In matters of the heart, processed meat is a bit scary because of two things, the shocking amount of sodium and the foreboding amount of fat and saturated fat in many of these products. The following chart lists the eight common processed meats and the typical amount of sodium and fat they contribute per serving.

The Processed Meat Line-Up

Processed meat is usually red meat preserved via smoking, curing, or salting. Sadly, this popular meat group includes many favorite American foods and sandwich meats:

	Sodium (mg)	Fat (g)	Saturated fat (g)	Cholesterol
Bacon, 3 strips	575	10	3.2	27
Ham lunchmeat, 2 oz	739	5	1.7	32
Sausage, 2 oz	306	11.5	3.2	56
Hot dog, 45 grams	461	14	5.6	25
Bologna, 2 oz	417	14	5.3	34
Salami, 2 oz	218	17	6	57
Pepperoni, 2 oz	980	26	12	70
Pastrami, 3 oz	753	6	2.3	58

The Salad Dressing Aisle

Hopefully you all know that the dark green lettuce types tend to have the most of all those important nutrients and phytochemicals such as spinach, romaine, and chicory. You can also tip the nutrition scales by adding other nutrient-rich plant foods to your salad (such as kidney beans, carrot coins, broccoli, tomato, etc.)

Once you have built yourself a nutrient-rich salad, the trick is not to make it a high-fat side or main dish by drenching it with a high-fat dressing. Regular salad dressing, mayonnaise, cream cheese, butter, and other "extras" can pour on the calories and saturated fat. If you aren't so sure if salad dressing should be grouped with other high fat items like butter or mayonnaise, this might convince you:

- Just 2 tablespoons of Girard's Caesar dressing contains 150 calories and 15 grams of fat
- Just 2 tablespoons of Wishbone Chunky Blue Cheese contains 160 calories and 17 grams of fat
- Just 2 tablespoons of Hidden Valley Ranch contains 140 calories and 14 grams of fat

The oil-and-vinegar-based dressings are, for the most part, going to have the nutritional advantage. A recent scientific analysis of plant foods and the prevention of cardiovascular disease noted that in the Nurses' Health Study, women who consumed oil-and-vinegar salad dressing frequently (greater than or equal to 5 to 6 times/week) had a 50 percent lower fatal coronary artery disease risk than those who rarely consumed this type of salad dressing. This association persisted even after the researchers adjusted for cardiovascular disease risk factors and the intake of vegetables.

When reading the labels, you'll find creamy and vinaigrette dressings that contain 8 grams or less of fat per 2 tablespoons and some with twice that amount. If you choose dressings that contain canola or olive oil, you will be getting the more protective monounsaturated fat, and in the case of canola oil, more plant omega-3s as well.

Choosing the right salad dressing is only half of the battle. Most people really need to pay attention to the amount of dressing, too. The serving size on the label of that bottle of salad dressing may say 2 tablespoons, but lots of people really add twice that amount. If you are eating out and you order your dressing on the side, use the small spoon and measure about 3 of those over your salad. This will get you about 1 1/2 tablespoons of dressing.

Cookie, Cracker, and Chip Aisles

For chips, it's all about the type and amount of oil used to make the chips. Most of the oils used to make chips are high in omega-6 fatty acids. Regular potato chips and Fritos tend to have about 10 grams of fat and 1 gram of saturated fat per ounce, while regular tortilla chips tend to have about 7 grams of fat per ounce, Which brings me to the fact that one ounce, the serving size on the bag, gets you only eight Tostito Multigrain chips or 12 Ruffles chips. If you are realistically eating twice that amount of chips (easy to do if you are eating them straight from a bag or bowl), then you need to double the nutritional damage. The calories increase to about 300 and the fat increases to about 20 grams of fat.

For tortilla chips, you can choose a brand with the least amount of fat (and/or one that uses a smart fat) that still tastes great, like Baked Doritos. For potato chips, you can find a lower fat alternative that you still enjoy such as Sun Chips with 6 grams of fat and 140 calories or Reduced Fat Ruffles with 7 grams fat. If you want to take it one step beyond that, there is Baked Ruffles (in several flavor options) with 3 grams fat and 120 calories per ounce. If you are Cheetos type of snacker, Baked Cheetos might satisfy your bright orange desire with 130 calories and 5 grams of fat per ounce.

Portion Tip: Grab a handful (usually works out to be about 1-ounce) and enjoy chips with your sandwich or small sirloin burger and fruit salad. You'll be more likely to be satisfied with 1 ounce this way.

When it comes to crackers, be careful reading nutrition information labels because some cracker brands use 1/2-ounce as the serving for the nutrition information label while others use 1 ounce. Most of the crackers on the market have about 6 to 8 grams of fat, 1 to 2 grams of saturated fat, and 200-300 mg sodium per 1-ounce serving (10 Ritz crackers, eight Keebler Club crackers, 27 Cheez-It crackers, etc.)

There used to be some trans fats lurking in the cracker aisle, but many manufacturers seem to have traded partially hydrogenated oils for palm oil (which naturally contributes some saturated fat). You'll find cracker options with more whole grain (and fiber) and some with less fat or less sodium...but you rarely find all three of these in the same cracker. These are some of the crackers I liked because they contribute some fiber without adding as much saturated fat and total fat as the average cracker.

1-Ounce Serving	Calories	Total Fat (g)	Saturated Fat (g)	Fiber (g)	Sodium (mg)
Nabisco Wheat Thins Fiber Selects 5-Grain crackers	120	4.5	.5	5	260
Triscuit Reduced Fat	120	3	.5	3	160
Ry Krisp New York Deli Rye	120	4	0	4	280

Trader Joe's Reduced Guilt Woven Wheats Wafers	120	2.5	0	3	210
Kashi TLC (tasty little crackers)	130	3	0	2	160

You know that yummy chocolate coating that's on certain cookies? That used to be a red flag warning that you were about to consume partially hydrogenated oils and therefore trans fat. Some of the brands have switched to using palm, coconut, or palm kernel oil, which may very well be non-hydrogenated oils, but they are also naturally saturated. Others are still using hydrogenated oils. This aisle is probably the last hold out for hydrogenated fat.

The Breakfast Cereal Aisle

Choosing a healthy breakfast cereal is not a simple task. The cereal aisle is a long one with a range of choices. You'll find cereals made with refined grains with nearly no fiber, and cereals made with whole grains and bran boasting 7 grams or more of fiber. There are cereals with so much sugar they seem more like boxes of little cookies. And there are cereals with sugar listed far down on the ingredient list.

Recent research suggests those who eat more whole grains are at lower risk of diabetes and heart disease.

The trick is finding a breakfast cereal that is full of healthful attributes, low in sugar, and has no saturated fat and trans fat, but still tastes great. It doesn't matter how good for you a cereal is; if it doesn't taste good, you're probably not going to eat it day after day. Of course, one person's perfect whole-grain cereal with less sugar is another person's bowl of sawdust.

The following cereals had an "excellent" or "very good" sensory rating, according to Consumer Reports, October 2009. Each of these seven top-rated cereals has at least 7 grams of fiber and the amount of sugar ranges from almost none (Shredded Wheat) to 18 grams per serving (Great Value Raisin Brain—the grams of sugar include the raisins).

	Fiber (g)	Sugars (g)	Calories	Sodium (mgs)
Excellent Sensory Rating				
Kirkland Signature Spiced Pecan (Costco), 3/4 cup	7	11	190	100
Very Good Sensory Rating				
Kashi GoLean Crunchy Fiber Twigs, Soy Protein Graham & Honey Puffs, 1 cup	10	6	140	85
Archer Farms High Fiber (Target), 1 cup	10	14	150	90
Kellogg's Raisin Bran Extra!, 1 cup	7	13	190	350
Post Shredded Wheat Spoon Size Wheat 'n Bran, 1 1/4 cup	8	<1	200	0

Great Value Raisin Bran (Wal-Mart), 1 cup	7	18	210	350
Barbara's Bakery Ultima Organic, 1 cup	12	9	170	280

The Produce Section

Finally, a section where pretty much anything goes! We should be eating fruits and vegetables at every single meal.

Sources

Djousse, L., et al. "Egg consumption in relation to cardiovascular disease and mortality: the Physicians' Health Study." *The American Journal of Clinical Nutrition* 87:4 (2008): 964–969.

Eckel, R.H. "Egg consumption in relation to cardiovascular disease and mortality: the story gets more complex." *The American Journal of Clinical Nutrition* 87:4 (2008): 799–800.

Oureshi, Al et al. "Regular egg consumption does not increase the risk of stroke and cardiovascular diseases."*Medical Science Monitor*. 13:1 (2007).

Hu, F.B. et al. "A Prospective Study of Egg Consumption and Risk of Cardiovascular Disease in Men and Women."*Journal of the American Medical Association*. 281:15 (1999): 1387–1394.

"Foods with More for Less: Rich in Nutrients, Low in Calories" *Environmental Nutrition* Feb 2008.

ESHA Research, Food Processor SQL, 2008 (nutrition analysis software)

Sinha R, et al. *Archives of Internal Medicine* 169:6 (2009): 562–571.

Fung T.T., Malik V., Rexrode, K.M., et al. "Sweetened beverage consumption and risk of coronary heart disease in women." *American Journal of Clinical Nutrition* 89:4 (2009): 1037–1042.

Steinke, L. "Effect of "Energy Drink" Consumption on Hemodynamic and Electrocardiographic Parameters in Healthy Young Adults." *Annals of Pharmacotherapy.* 43:4 (2009): 596–602.

Dhingra, R., Sullivan, L., Jacques, PF, et al. "Soft Drink Consumption and Risk of Developing Cardiometabolic Risk Factors and the Metabolic Syndrome in Middle Aged Adults in the Community." *Circulation* 116 (2007): 1–9.

"Statement of American Beverage Association Regarding Soft Drink Consumption Study in Circulation." *American Beverage Association* 23 Jul 2007.

Iqbal, R., Anand, S., Ounpuu, S. et al. "Dietary Patterns and the Risk of Acute Myocardial Infarction in 52 Countries." *Circulation* 118 (2008): 1929–1937.

How Not to Eat Your Heart Out When Eating Out

For most of us, the mere act of eating in restaurants somehow puts us in "splurge" mode. We eat foods that are rich and that we wouldn't normally eat, and we finish the large portions that we're served. To counter this, we should do the exact opposite.

Key #1: Make better food choices.

Restaurant menu items are usually high in the items we are trying to eat less of: calories, fat, saturated fat (some restaurants and fast food chains are still using fats with trans fat), cholesterol, and sodium. The biggest challenge? We usually have no idea how many calories or grams of saturated fat are in the menu items. Perhaps if we knew, we would make different selections or at the very least we would try hard not to overeat or order calorie-containing drinks and desserts.

Key #2: Make "moderation" your eating-out mantra.

Restaurants tend to serve it up in huge portions, and studies suggest that the more food we are served, the more food we tend to eat. The type of food served by restaurants and fast-food chains encourages overeating because the food is typically lower in the things that help us feel full and satisfied (such as fiber and water). Eating meals that include deep-fried foods, refined grains, and sweetened beverages appears to chemically encourage us to eat more food. All of these factors are at play when eating out, creating the "perfect storm" that affects heart health and losing weight.

Key #3: Make trips to fast-food restaurants occasionally, not daily.

Frequenting the drive-through is an unavoidable part of modern life, but keep it to an occasional dalliance.

10 Heart-Healthy Restaurant Tips

1. Go for beverages with zero calories.

2. Downsize your portions, and eat slowly so you enjoy each bite. You'll be more likely to feel satisfied sooner.

3. Ask how a particular dish is prepared. In many cases, it can be prepared differently—meaning, instead of frying the fish, it could be grilled.

4. Look for opportunities to order menu items that include high nutrients and high-fiber fruits, vegetables, and beans.

5. Opt for condiments that contribute less than 25 calories per serving (such as ketchup, mustard, or marinara or barbecue sauce). Or opt for condiments that feature smart fats like avocado slices or olive oil–based pesto sauce.

6. Make a point of enjoying fish (not deep-fried) when in restaurants. This is a great way to get your weekly dose of fish and their awesome omega-3 fatty acids.

7. Calories and extra fat from appetizers and table munchies add up fast. Don't over-order just because you're super hungry.

8. Salt (or sodium-containing sauce) is already added to most food prepared in restaurants. So think long and hard before reaching for that salt shaker.

9. Order your dessert with extra forks, and share it with everyone at the table. The first few bites are usually the best anyway.

10. Look for nutritional information about what you're ordering whenever possible. Most of us go to the same fast-food chains over and over, and most of those chains have Websites that offer nutritional information about their menus. Check out the items you are interested in, and see which ones are lowest in the things we're trying to eat less of (calories, saturated and trans fat, sodium, and total fat).

    As for restaurants, many chains have nutritional information available as a separate menu, with precious few offering the information on their Websites. If the restaurant doesn't provide these numbers, pay attention to how the selection is described on the menu. Words like flaky, pastry, fritters, breaded and fried, deep-fried, cream sauce, buttery, and crispy usually describe higher fat and calorie choices. Words such as grilled, steamed, poached, tomato- or broth-based, whole grains, beans, fish, skinless poultry, stir-fry, or olive oil will guide you to higher fiber and lower saturated fat choices.

Fast Food's Worst Trans Fat Offenders

Trans fats are still lurking in some fast food, and that's bad. But what's also alarming is that many of the items that used to be the worst in trans fat are now the worst in saturated fat. Chains have traded saturated fat for the trans fat they have taken out, so make sure you consider both numbers when you are looking up the nutrition information online.

The American Heart Association advises Americans to consume no more than 2 grams of trans fat per day. Two grams a day? That's definitely a best-case scenario. In today's food world, it's easier than you think to eat double or triple the daily 2-gram goal in just one meal, especially if you frequent certain fast-food chains.

Looking through this nutritional information, I uncovered a few trans fat truths:

- Trans fat used to be hiding in pastries, pie crusts, and biscuits.
- Breaded and fried chicken and seafood can contribute more trans fat than you think.
- Trans fat can even be lurking in full-fat dairy and beef selections.
- Certain fast-food chains still use cooking fats that have trans fats—meaning your favorite fries might be cooked in them.
- Some fast-food desserts carry a few grams of trans fat as well.

Index

About the Author

Elaine Magee is passionate about changing the way America eats—one recipe at a time! She is the author of the celebrated syndicated column "The Recipe Doctor" and has contributed recipes to multiple Websites and magazines. Her personal Website is *www.recipedoctor.com*. Magee is a nutrition expert for WebMD and a frequent guest on TV and radio shows across the country. She is the author of 25 previous books on nutrition and cooking, including *Food Synergy*, as well as other titles in the *Tell Me What To Eat* series, covering diabetes, acid reflux disease, Irritable Bowel Syndrome, menopause, colon cancer, breast cancer, and headaches and migraines. She obtained her Master's Degree in public health nutrition from UC-Berkeley and is a registered dietitian.